VACCINE DELIVERY AND AUTISM

THE LATEX CONNECTION

Michael J. Dochniak
Denise H. Dunn

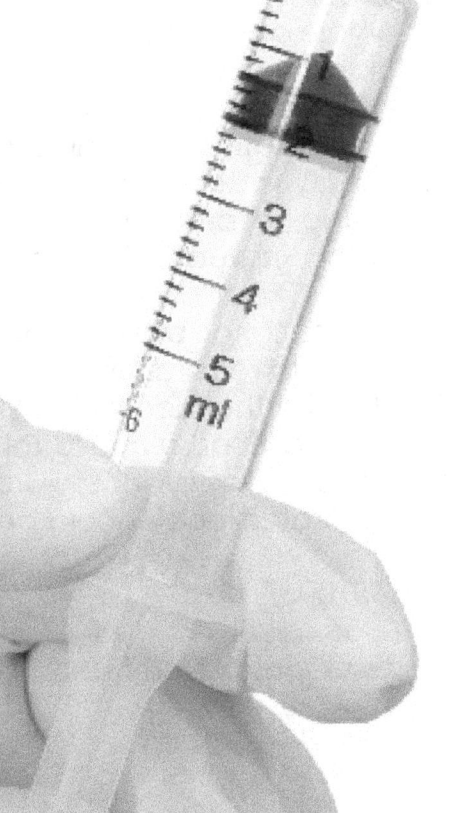

Michael J. Dochniak
Telephone 612-836-8237
E-mail: mdochniak@yahoo.com

Notice to the reader: The authors have taken special care in the preparation of this book, but make no expressed or implied warranty of any kind and assume no responsibility for any errors or omissions. No liability is assumed for incidental or consequential damages in connection with or arising out of information contained in this book. The authors shall not be liable for any special, consequential, or exemplary damages resulting, in whole or in part, from the readers' use of, or reliance upon, this material.

Independent verification should be sought for any data, advice or recommendations contained in this book. In addition, no responsibility is assumed by the authors for any injury and/or damage to persons or property arising from any method, products, instructions, ideas, or otherwise contained in this book.

This book is designed to provide accurate and authoritative information with regard to the subject matter covered herein. It is sold with the clear understanding that the authors are not engaged in rendering legal or any other professional services. If legal assistance is required, the services of a recognized professional should be sought.

ISBN-13: 978-1456570057
ISBN-10: 1456570056
Library of Congress Control Number: 2011901310

———

Dedication

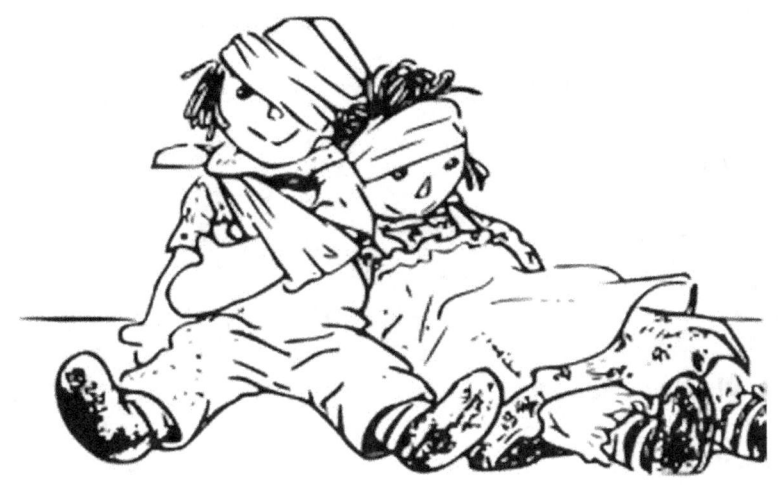

Raggedy Ann and Andy

To individuals permanently harmed by vaccinations

To individuals who seek to answer the question:

Is allergy-induced regressive autism
caused by vaccinations?

We Honor You

———

To Harmony Dunn, you're inspirational, compassionate, insightful, and creative; making this book possible.

———

Table of Contents

———

Preface

Vaccination and childhood regression increasing each year
Medical science makes it clear
Vaccine be disarmed
Protein contamination can harm
Allergens in rubber diffuse
Adjuvants seduce
Adaptive immunity deduce
Atopy will produce...
Allergy-induced regressive autism

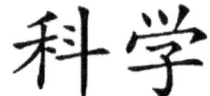

Science

—

Welcome,

Autism rates have risen sharply. I want everyone to know that the story of allergy-induced regressive autism is a hopeful journey. It shows us we can walk on a meaningful path of natural-latex allergy prevention.

I believe that *Hevea brasiliensis* dry natural-rubber (*HDNR*) exclusionary practice and ultra-low protein natural latex will show us that when exposure to the *Hevea*-allergens is eliminated, the incidence of atopy and allergy-induced regressive autism will diminish in successive generations.

Over the years, I've learned much about how *HDNR* can affect our lives in very different ways. For most, *HDNR* is a material that contributes to a better standard of living, while for others, exposure can be harmful and even life threatening. I also support the idea that in many rubber applications, it's naïve to believe that *HDNR* can be completely replaced with synthetic rubber; natural latex has a price/performance characteristic that continues to be second to none. Because of this, every effort should be made to substantially remove the allergens from HDNR. Although in medical applications, including vaccines, HDNR should not be used, as the allergens can never be completely removed.

I think that vaccines contributed to my son's regressive autism and this book will show how the HDNR used in vaccines, paired with atypical adaptive immunity, can cause allergy-induced regressive autism.

HDNR in vaccines violate the first rule of medicine: "Do no harm."

Sincerely,
Michael J. Dochniak

Dear Reader,

Vaccines clearly affected my son's immunity and personality. As a parent, I resisted vaccinating my child and he met developmental milestones. During adolescence, I reluctantly had him vaccinated. Shortly thereafter, he developed food sensitivity and atypical behaviors. At the same time, he developed fractured skills. He excelled in deductive reasoning and paradigm thinking but regressed in emotional development and social interaction. After three years of intervention including disciplinary probation, social training, medical and educational support, he was diagnosed with Aspergers Syndrome by a Pediatric Neuropsychologist.

Vaccine safety is critical and it should be a never-ending process. Learn how vital it is for immune-sensitive children to be protected from vaccine insult.

Sincerely,
Harmony Dunn

———

Introduction

Fringe science is a flavor of conjecture
Conjecture is an ingredient of creativity
Creativity is a recipe for hypotheses
A hypothesis feeds medical science
Medical science then nourishes mankind
Knowledge grows

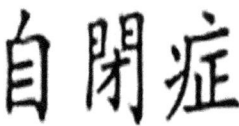

Autism

———

Can vaccines cause autism?

The chronology below exemplifies the uncertainty, complexity, and urgency of this question.

(1998)   Dr. Andrew Wakefield called for a suspension of the measles, mumps and rubella (MMR) vaccine until more research could be done. Dr. Wakefield was a British surgeon and is a researcher known for his work regarding the MMR vaccine and its possible connection with autism and inflammatory bowel disease.

(2009)   The director of the National Institute of Neurological Disorders and Stroke (NINDS) stated that autism researchers should study "the children who have been most profoundly affected" by adverse reactions to vaccination.

(2009)   The American Medical Association (AMA) rejected a call for more research on a vaccine link to autism, and reaffirmed immunization policies. California delegate and internist Melvyn Sterling, M.D., testified during a reference committee hearing that sufficient research on vaccines and autism already exists and clearly demonstrates the two are not linked.

(2009)   Paul A. Offit of Children's Hospital of Philadelphia wrote, "When one hypothesis of how vaccines cause autism is refuted, another invariably springs up to take its place." Dr. Offit is a member of the Centers for Disease Control (CDC) Advisory Committee on Immunization Practices and author of the book titled, *Autism's False Prophets: Bad Science, Risky Medicine, and the Search for a Cure.*

(2009)   The U.S. Court of Appeals for the Federal Circuit upheld a ruling of a special vaccine court denying a link between vaccines and autism. The "vaccines court" ruled in three separate cases that the mercury-containing preservative Thimerosal does not cause autism.

(2010)   *The Lancet* retracted a medical-journal paper by Dr. Wakefield et al. linking vaccines to autism. The retraction states, "The claims in the original paper that children were 'consecutively referred' and that investigations were 'approved' by the local ethics committee have been proven to be false."

(2010)   A U.S. court rules that vaccines' containing a mercury-based preservative called Thimerosal does not cause autism on their own.

(2010)   A study published in the journal *Pediatrics* showed that one in four parents is concerned that vaccines can cause autism.

The CDC continues to state that, "Vaccines are developed with the highest standards of safety. However, as with any medical procedure, vaccination has some risks. Individuals react differently to vaccines, and there is no way to predict how individuals will react to a particular vaccine."

There are many factors that can affect how our bodies react to a vaccine. In this book, the authors use empirical evidence, anecdotal evidence, and scientific reasoning to show that allergens (i.e., environmental insult) from HDNR can contaminate vaccines causing atopy and allergy-induced regressive autism in some children.

Briefly, there are primarily two types of immunity;

Innate immunity - The antibodies immunoglobulin-G (IgG) and immunoglobulin-M (IgM), protect us from being harmed by infectious microorganisms, these are referred to as innate immunity; and

Adaptive immunity - Immunoglobulin-E (IgE) antibodies help defend against viral and bacterial infection, destroy parasites, and capture non-infectious proteins called allergens, which cause allergies and possibly atopy.

Atopy is a disease characterized by a tendency to be "hyper-allergic" (i.e., have multiple allergies). Atopy is a word taken from the Greek meaning "special" or "unusual." Many physicians and scientists use the term atopy for any IgE antibody-mediated reaction. Other pediatricians reserve the word atopy for a genetically-mediated predisposition to an excessive IgE reaction, but environmental factors are also suspected to play a major role in atopy. Research indicates that atopy plays a role in the etiology of regressive autism.

Regressive autism occurs when a child appears to develop typically but then starts to lose speech and social skills, usually between the ages of fifteen and thirty months, and is subsequently diagnosed with autism.

How can we explain and respond to the rapid increase of autism spectrum disorders?

According to Autism Speaks, a non-profit public awareness organization, it is estimated today that one in every 110 children is diagnosed with autism, making it more common than childhood cancer, juvenile diabetes, and pediatric AIDS combined. An estimated 1.5 million individuals in the United States and tens of millions worldwide are affected.

Government statistics suggest the prevalence rate of autism is increasing 10 to 17 percent annually. While the causes of autism are complex and puzzling, a consensus is emerging that atypical immunity likely plays a dominant role.

This book provides a fresh look at autism, which is one of the most perplexing scientific and medical questions of our time. The authors clearly show that HDNR, which continues to be a part of some vaccines, can adversely affect adaptive immunity; increasing the incidence of atopy and allergy-induced regressive autism.

What if...

- parents start refusing vaccines that contain HDNR to help reduce latex allergy?
- pharmaceutical companies practiced HDNR exclusion to help reduce latex allergy?
- the U.S. government regulated the protein content of HDNR to help reduce latex allergy?
- physicians' implemented blood screening tests to help reduce vaccine related injuries?

In summary, increased HDNR exposure and sensitivity is likely associated with the steep rise in atopy and allergy-induced regressive autism over the last thirty years. In the future, we need to make sure vaccines are free of HDNR.

"I continue to fully support more independent research to determine if environmental triggers, including vaccines, are causing autism and other developmental problems. The current rate of autism is 1 in 110 children in the United States and 1 in 64 children in the U.K. My goal has always been and will remain the health and safety of children. Since the Lancet paper, I have lost my job, my career and my country. To claim that my motivation was profit is patently untrue. I will not be deterred - this issue is far too important."
- Andrew J. Wakefield (Autism Researcher)

———

1

Chapter 1

Natural-latex, powdered glove, barrier supreme
Feeling protected but rash in hand
Powder inhaled and breath assailed
Lungs can't expand
Asthma firsthand

~

Dry natural latex in vaccine packaging and delivery
Harmful protein-contamination danger foreseen
Adaptive immunity often unseen
Allergy-induced regressive autism not serene

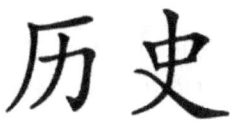

History

———

Medical History

Natural latex has a long history. The first was by the Olmecs, who centuries later passed on the knowledge of this material to the ancient Mayans.[1] The chronology below exemplifies a brief medical history of natural latex.

(1894)   William Stewart Halsted, the first surgeon in chief at Johns Hopkins Hospital, was widely credited as the pioneer who developed and introduced natural-latex surgical gloves into the United States.[2]

(1927)   Descriptions of allergic reactions to natural latex started to appear in the medical literature.[3]

(1979)   Immediate-type allergic reactions from natural-latex exposure were first reported.[4]

(1984)   Anaphylactic reactions caused by natural-latex surgical gloves were reported.[5]

(1991)   Reports of fatal anaphylactic reactions to natural-latex surgical gloves.[6]

(1993)   Irritant and delayed-contact reactions from natural latex were documented in a medical paper entitled, "Is Cow's Milk Casein an Allergen in Latex-Rubber Gloves?"[7]

(1998)   The FDA added a warning on medical devices containing natural latex.[8]

(2008)   Natural latex is banned at Johns Hopkins Hospital.[9]

(2010)   Nova Science published a book entitled, *Allergies and Autism* that describes how the antigenic proteins in natural latex affect the incidence of atopy and allergy-induced regressive autism.[10]

(2010)   *The Journal of Molecular Neuroscience* published, "A Proteomic Investigation of B Lymphocytes in an Autistic Family: A Pilot Study of Exposure to Natural rubber latex (NRL) May Lead to Autism." [11]

(2010)   The FDA required label changes for flu vaccines to highlight natural-latex concerns.[12]

As described above, hospitals are just beginning to eliminate natural latex in their facilities because of a dramatic increase in latex allergies. It is important for consumers to known that some vaccines still contain natural latex in their packaging and delivery system (e.g., vial stoppers or seals and syringe plungers). It is suspected that mass vaccination campaigns continue to increases latex allergy.

How many vaccines do children receive?

The chronology below presents the frequency of childhood vaccines before entering school.

(1960)   Children received 1 or 2 vaccines.
(1980)   Children were routinely given 8 to 9 vaccines.
(1990)   Children received about 10 vaccinations.
(2010)   Children were routinely given about 33 vaccinations.[13]

In clarification, the term "latex" has often been used to describe natural latex, causing some confusion; synthetic polymers are also referred to as "latex". In response the U.S. Food and Drug Administration, which is emboldened to protect the health and safety of all Americans, has clarified the latex-terminology associated with natural latex as follows:

- Natural latex (NL) is defined as a milky fluid that consists of extremely small particles of rubber obtained from a rubber tree. It contains a variety of substances and plant proteins thought to be primary allergens;
- Natural rubber (NR) includes all materials made from or containing natural latex. Natural-rubber-containing

products are made using two common processes: the Natural-Rubber-Latex (NRL) liquid process and the Dry-Natural-Rubber (DNR or *HDNR*) process; and

- The phrase "contains natural rubber" includes NRL and DNR products as well as any synthetic latex or synthetic rubbers that contain natural rubber. This definition does not include any synthetic latex or synthetic rubber product that contains no natural rubber.

I have a terrible latex allergy; it actually blisters and burns my skin off. If it got into my bloodstream, it would probably kill me. – Andiarose, WrongPlanet.Net, Women's Discussion

———

Notes

1. "Natural Rubber," Wikipedia, The free encyclopedia, http://en.wikipedia.org/wiki/Natural_rubber, accessed 1/11/11.
2. Eric Vohr, "Rubber Gloves 'Born'- and Now Banished- at Johns Hopkins," *The JHU Gazette* 37, 18 (2008), http://www.jhu.edu/~gazette/2008/22jan08/22gloves.html, accessed 1/11/11.
3. Stern J. Ueberempfindlichkeit gegen Kautschuk als Ursache von Urticaria und Quinkeschem Oedem Klin Wochenschr 1927; 6; 1479.
4. A. Nutter, "Contact Urticaria to Rubber: *Br. J. Dermatology* 101 (1979): 597-8, http://www.ncbi.nlm.nih.gov/pubmed/518831?dopt=Abstract, accessed 1/11/11.
5. S.S. Entman and K.J. Moise, "Anaphylaxis in Pregnancy," *South Med. J.* 77 (1984): 402, accessed 1/11/11, http://www.ncbi.nlm.nih.gov/pubmed/6701631, accessed 1/11/11.
6. Ownby et al., "Anaphylaxis Associated with Latex Allergy During Barium Enema Examinations," *Am. J. Roentgenol* 156 (1991):903-8.

7. S. Makinen-Kiljunen, T. Reunala, K. Turjanmaa, and P. Cacioli, "Is Cow's Milk Casein an Allergen in Latex-Rubber Gloves," *Lancet* 342 (1993):863-4.

8. Health Publications, "Final rule adds warning on devices containing latex,' http://findarticles. com/p/articles/mi_m1370/is_n1_v32/ai_20356435/, accessed 1/11/11.

9. Physorg.com, "Latex Banned at Johns Hopkins Hospital," January 18, 2008, http://www.physorg. com/news119886779.html, accessed 1/11/11.

10. M.J. Dochniak, D.H. Dunn, *Allergies and Autism*, Allergies and Infectious Diseases Series (NY: Nova Science Publishers, 2010).

11. C. Shen, et al., "A Proteomic Investigation of B Lymphocytes In an Autistic Family: A Pilot Study of Exposure to Natural Rubber Latex (NRL) May Lead to Autism," *J. Mol. Neurosci.* (2010).

12. American Academy of Family Physicians, AAFP, News Now, "FDA Requires Label Changes for Flu Vaccines to Highlight Latex Concerns," http://www.aafp.org/online/en/home/ publications/news/news-now/clinical-care-research/20100825fluvaccinelatex.html, accessed 1/11/11.

13. CDC, "Recommended Immunization Schedule," http://www.cdc.gov/vaccines/recs/schedules/ downloads/child/2010/10_0-6yrs_chart_only.jpg, accessed 1/11/11.

———

2

Chapter 2

Dry natural rubber, part of vaccines
Cut, slash, gather, and collect what bleeds
Milky-white colloid from Para Rubber Tree
Latex allergy, mankind beware
Harmful allergens, Doctors take care
Nurses and Parents make sure it's not there

~

Government involvement
It's only fair
FDA, CDC, NVPO standards...
Let's make aware

~

Dry natural rubber
Take out of vaccines
It's not safe, and it's not clean

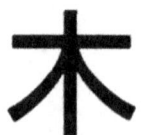

Tree

—

Natural latex

One of the best-known "natural" polymers is polyisoprene. Ancient Mayans and Aztecs, in what is now Central America, harvested it from the *Hevea brasiliensis* tree to make waterproof boots, containers, and balls that they used to play a game similar to basketball. In the Amazon, the *Hevea brasiliensis* tree was known as the weeping tree, the white blood of the forest. For generations, Indians slashed its bark, letting the latex drip onto leaves, where it could be molded by hand into vessels and sheets that were impermeable to the rain.

NRL, the milky-white colloid tapped from the *Hevea brasiliensis* rubber tree, has been used for thousands of years and, today, can be found in over forty thousand products. NRL continues to be produced by a process wherein the rubber tree is cut or slashed, using a knife or machete, through the bark, wounding the tree. The NRL bleeds from the wound and is collected in a reservoir such as a coconut cup. Thereafter, the NRL is dehydrated to form *HDNR* and vulcanized. Vulcanization is a process of treating natural latex with sulfur and then using heat and pressure to improve its elasticity and strength.

HDNR is produced primarily in a dozen tropical countries, including Thailand, Indonesia, Malaysia, Vietnam, Liberia, and India. The overwhelming (approximately 90%) volume of natural latex comes from *Hevea brasiliensis*. It is estimated that global natural-latex production is about 22.2 billion pounds each year.[1]

Natural latex has been the material of choice in the medical industry due to its unique properties, including sealing properties, self-sealing properties, chemical resistance, and stability after sterilization. The material within natural latex that gives rubber its useful properties is the polymer called polyisoprene. The polyisoprene found in natural latex does not cause the allergic reactions. Reactions are caused by the allergenic or antigenic proteins in natural latex.

There are approximately two hundred or more dissimilar proteins in HDNR; about 2 to 5 percent based on the total weight. Of these proteins, fifty to sixty are suspected allergens. The World Health Organization (WHO) has assigned names to thirteen of these proteins that have been shown to cause latex allergy.

Allergies of all kinds affect over fifty million people in the United States. Within the overall population of individuals with allergies, a significant number has "latex allergy." Studies on the prevalence of latex allergy in sera of blood donors in the United States and Europe vary from 4.6 percent to7.6 percent.[2]

It is speculated that repeated exposure to natural latex has caused a global increase in allergies, especially in industrialized societies. HDNR contains a plethora of proteins (i.e., Hevea-allergens), which are known to have structural homology to beneficial proteins. For example, it is well known that the Hevea-allergens can confuse the adaptive immune system, causing increased sensitivity to food proteins.

The health and safety issues associated with the Hevea-allergens continue to affect medical industry policies and practices. For example, John Hopkins researchers have encouraged the Food and Drug Administration (FDA) and pharmaceutical companies to discontinue the use of natural latex for stoppers in medical vials.[3]

There are alternative materials, although more expensive, that can be used to replace natural latex (e.g., silicone rubber) in vaccines.

Although Hevea-allergen petitions and warnings have been documented, in 2006, the United States Safety Commission denied petition HP-002 requesting a rule declaring HDNR to be a strong sensitizer. However, the Honorable Thomas H. Moore (Commissioner) stated, "Nevertheless, it would behoove manufacturers of NRL to take steps to reduce the level of proteins that consumers can come into contact with, whether or not the end product is a medical device."[4]

The medical profession now recognizes the hazards of *Hevea-brasiliensis* NRL. In 2008, Johns Hopkins Hospital banned nearly all natural-latex products.[5]

Why are the *Hevea*-allergens dangerous?

Exposure to the *Hevea*-allergens through inhalation, dermal contact, sublingual absorption, and vaccine injection has been shown to cause an increased incidence of sensitization, adverse allergic reactions, and even death through anaphylactic shock. For example, health care workers, using natural-latex gloves in an attempt to reduce the accidental spread of viral infections including Autoimmune Deficiency Syndrome (AIDS), have experienced an increased number of sensitizations and death from these gloves. Because of such medical-worker-exposure data, HDNR is recognized as a hazardous material by the National Institute for Occupational Safety and Health.[6]

Furthermore, latex allergy may be a catalyst for the onset of food allergies. What can be perplexing is that latex allergy can go into remission from reduced exposure, while subsequent food allergies may remain persistent based on repeated exposure to such food proteins. Thus, the after effects of latex allergy may continue to stress adaptive immunity long after the latex allergy has gone into remission. In fact, one study showed that almost 50 percent of patients with natural-latex allergy showed food allergies.[7]

The incidence of natural-latex allergy continues to be monitored and researched. Not surprisingly, the prevalence of latex allergy continues to rise. In a study on natural-latex-specific IgE from patients at an urban hospital emergency room, data showed that the overall percentage of seropositive for latex-specific IgE was 8.2 percent. The researchers concluded that the prevalence of Natural-latex sensitization in their sampling is substantial and higher than previously estimated in the general adult population (i.e., 1 percent to 5 percent).[8]

It is well known that the natural latex used in vaccines can be harmful. For example, in a case report on natural-latex hypersensitivity, it was determined that a diabetic six-year-old girl was constantly exposed to small amounts of natural latex through the plungers in insulin syringes and the stoppers in insulin vials. The physician reported that she had no physical reactions to the insulin shots but was frightened and tearful prior to injection. The family began noticing skin reactions at the site of the injections after most but not all injections. The reactions were described as red and blotchy and were said to be between the sizes of a dime and nickel (1-1.5 cm). They were swollen and pruritic for about two to three hours after the injection. The reactions lasted up to twenty-four hours. Her mother at this time also began noting a similar type of reaction with the use of adhesive bandages. Intradermal testing verified latex allergy. The physician learned that the septum in the insulin vial was made of hardened natural latex made from harvested *Hevea brasiliensis*. Latex avoidance procedures were implemented quickly and effectively to help reduce the frequency of such reactions.[9]

Government agencies, including the FDA and Centers for Disease Control and Prevention (CDC), continue to warn industry and consumers about the hazards of HDNR used in some vaccines. Unfortunately, the threshold of sensitivity and severity of reactions to the *Hevea*-allergens is unknown based on the unpredictable characteristic of adaptive immunity. Therefore, even minute quantities in vaccines (e.g., parts per billion) could trigger sensitivity or an adverse allergic reaction.

In the spirit of "do not harm," it is the opinion of the authors that HDNR needs to be discontinued for use in vaccines, knowing that the *Hevea*-allergens are ever-present.

The stress-strain curves from Hevea brasiliensis *dry natural rubber continue to stretch the imagination.* – Michael J. Dochniak

———

Notes

1. Rubbernews.com, http://www.rubbernews.com/subscriber/morenews.html, accessed 1/11/11.
2. Dudek, et al., "Natural Rubber Latex Allergy: Antigen Specific IgE in Polish Blood Donors, Prevalence and Risk Factors – Preliminary Data," *International Journal of Occupational Medicine and Environmental Health*, 18, 1 (2005):35-42.
3. Kate O' Rourke, "Drug Bottles Containing Natural Rubber Stoppers May Place Latex Allergic Patients at Risk for reactions: Hopkins Researchers Encourage FDA and Pharmaceutical Companies to End Natural Rubber Stopper Use," June 8, 2001, http://www.hopkinsmedicine.org/press/2001/June/010608.htm, accessed 1/11/11.
4. Todd Stevens, Citizen Petition HP00-2, Requesting a Rule Declaring Natural Rubber Latex to be a Strong Sensitizer, April 30th, U.S. Consumer Product Safety Commission, deposition HP00-2, 2004.
5. Physorg.com, "Latex Banned at Johns Hopkins Hospital," January 18, 2008, http://www.physorg.com/news119886779.html, accessed 1/11/11.
6. NIOSH Publication NO. 97-135, "Preventing Allergic Reactions to Natural Rubber Latex in the Workplace," June 1997, http://www.cdc.gov/niosh/latex alt.html, accessed 1/11/11.
7. Carlos Blanco, "Latex-Fruit Syndrome," *Current Allergy and Asthma Reports* 3 (2003):47-53.
8. Mary Grzybowski et al., The Prevalence of Latex-Specific IgE In Patients Presenting to an Urban Emergency Department, *Annals of Emergency Medicine*, 40, 4 (2002):411-419.
9. Robert P. Hoffman, "Latex Hypersensitivity in a Child with Diabetes," *Arch. Pediatr. Adolesc. Med.* 154 (2000):281-282.

3

Chapter 3

Dry Natural Rubber
and
Vaccine Delivery
Hevea-allergens leach from stopper, it's improper
Vaccine injected…
Hevea-allergen antibodies to be found
Beneficial proteins can be bound
Cross-reactivity more and more around
Atopy profound

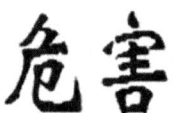

Harm

———

Hevea-allergen Antibodies

Antibodies developed from allergen exposure are most often IgE. The IgE are believed to have first evolved as a mechanism to protect mammals against parasites; however, in industrialized countries, allergens now represent a far greater threat than parasitic infection.

The *Hevea*-allergens have dramatically presented themselves over the last thirty years in medical products.

The WHO, International Union of Immunological Societies, has assigned names to thirteen of these allergens (Hev-b 1 to Hev-b 13).

Hevea-allergens are a complex mixture of antigenic proteins. It is recognized that some of these proteins are oil soluble (hydrophobic) while others are water soluble (hydrophilic). Furthermore, many of these allergens have variable degrees of cross-linking, molecular weight, and amino acid content. In summary, the Hevea-allergens are a botanical mixture of harmful antigenic-proteins that the immune system has to deal with.

Can Hevea-allergen contaminated vaccines induce atopy?

To answer this question, it's important to take a look at how the adaptive immune system recognizes and handles the Hevea-allergens.

It is generally understood that atopy may be acquired by excessive B-cell and T-cell production. Briefly, when B-cells and T-cells are activated after vaccination, some will become memory cells. If the vaccine is contaminated with Hevea-allergens, the immune system may produce allergen-specific memory cells to produce B and T lymphocytes affecting latex allergy.

Thereafter, newly encountered Hevea-allergens cause these memory cells to be selected and activated. In this manner, the second and subsequent exposures to Hevea-allergens produce a stronger and faster immune response. This is "adaptive" because the body's immune system prepares itself for future challenges.

It is important to note that the innate and adaptive portions of the immune system work together and not in spite of each other. The adaptive arm, B and T cells, would be unable to function without the input of the innate system. T-cells are useless without antigen-presenting cells to activate them, and B cells are crippled without T-cell help. Without this relationship, the innate system would likely be overrun with pathogens without the specialized action of the adaptive immune response.[1]

We know that the immune system is capable of producing more than one trillion different antibody molecules. Millions of genes would be required to store the genetic information used to produce these receptors, but the entire human genome contains fewer than twenty-five thousand genes. This myriad of receptors is produced through a process known as clonal selection According to the clonal selection theory; an infant will randomly generate a vast diversity of lymphocytes (each bearing a unique antigen receptor) from information encoded in a small family of genes. In order to generate each unique allergen receptor, these genes will have undergone a process called V(D)J recombination, or combinatorial diversification, in which one gene segment recombines with other gene segments to form a single unique gene. It is this assembly process that generates the enormous diversity of receptors and antibodies.

The structural complexity of the Hevea-allergens can confuse the immune system. Many of the allergens are large protein-molecules having unusual amino acid composition and sequence. The segments of the allergen that interact with an IgE are called epitopes. Thus, the Hevea-allergens contain many epitopes that can stimulate the production of a multiplicity of IgE and specific T-cell responses.

When an infant is insulted with a Hevea-allergen contaminated vaccine, the immune system is designed to "remember" and eliminate a large number of these allergens. Essentially, the immune system is forced to distinguish its many different epitopes. Furthermore, the receptors that recognize these allergens must be produced in a huge variety of configurations, essentially one receptor (at least) for each different Hevea-allergen that is encountered. Thus, the sheer number of antigenic proteins and epitope complexity associated with Hevea-allergens makes it a potentially dangerous material. Furthermore, because of the enormous diversity of Hevea-allergens, a vast quantity of IgE may be formed that can, through cross-reactivity, bind to beneficial proteins based on structure or epitope homology. It is well documented that latex allergy can cause cross-reactivity that perpetuates allergic responses (i.e., atopy) to beneficial proteins including food stuff proteins.[2]

Does atopy affect some of the symptoms associated with allergy-induced-regressive autism?

A study evaluated whether there is an association between atopic disorders and irritable bowel syndrome (IBS). The research showed that individuals with atopic symptoms report a higher incidence of IBS, suggesting a link between atopy and IBS.[3]

In an article published in *European Medical Device Technology* (EMDT) it is written, the release of allergenic proteins from the *HDNR* components of prefilled syringes into aqueous pharmaceuticals may potentially induce an immediate allergic reaction in individuals with a latex protein allergy. The article goes on to review the current risks to patients in the context of vaccine delivery. They concluded that all the data collected from the literature support the conclusion that exposure to *HDNR* components presents a residual health and hazard risk and that it is an acceptable risk considering the benefits of prefilled syringes for drug delivery.[4] It's apparent the medical community is presented with a conundrum when it comes to *HDNR* and vaccine safety.

Why is *HDNR* still used in vaccines?

The medical industry clearly recognizes that *Hevea*-allergen contamination in vaccines can be harmful. In support of this, the FDA requires natural-latex warning labels on vaccines that use *HDNR*. Unfortunately, consumers have no access to the latex warnings on vaccine packaging and vaccine delivery systems.

Hevea-allergens catalyze the sales of allergy medication. – Michael J. Dochniak

———

Notes

1. "Adaptive immune system," Wikipedia, The free encyclopedia, http://en.wikipedia.org/wiki/Adaptive_immune_system, accessed 1/11/11.
2. Tom Greer, Greer Laboratories Inc., "Literature Review on Latex-Food Cross-Reactivity 1991-2006," http://www.latexallergyresources.org/FileDownloads/Latex-food%20cross-reactivity%20review.pdf, accessed 111/11.
3. M.C. Tobin et al., "Atopic Irritable Bowel Syndrome; A Novel Subgroup of Irritable Bowel Syndrome with Allergic Manifestations," *Ann. Allergy Immunol.*, Jan, 100 (1), 49-53 (2008).
4. Philippe E. Laurent et al., "Dry Natural Rubber Components in Prefilled Syringes," *European Medical Device Technology*, 1, 3 (2010).

———

4

Chapter 4

Infectious organisms, present through time
Body is attacked
Immune cells react
Humans to live
Humans to die
When antibodies flourish, pathogens perish
Disease at ease
When antibodies fail, pathogens assail
Death will prevail
Pandemic not kind, infections change the mind
Neurotrophin expression
Sympathetic networks grow
Intelligence to know

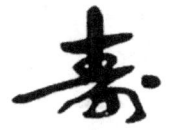

Long life
—

Life Design

An infinite number of the tiny organisms we call viruses and bacteria have and will continue to challenge our existence on this planet. By the toll of a billion deaths from infection, man has an immunity that is earned.

Have viruses, bacteria, and allergens played an essential role in the evolution of mankind?

Viruses are an important natural means of transferring genes between different species, thereby increasing genetic diversity and driving evolution. It is thought that viruses played a central role in the early evolution of life, before the diversification of bacteria, archaea, and eukaryotes and at the time of the last universal common ancestor of life on Earth. Viruses are still one of the largest reservoirs of unexplored genetic diversity on the Earth.[1]

Unfortunately, viruses can also be very destructive and have killed large segments of the population. A pandemic is an epidemic of infectious disease that spreads through human populations across a large region, such as a continent or even the entire world. The Influenza Epidemic of 1918-1919 erupted suddenly and unmercifully killed twenty million people. It has been suggested that those who were infected and survived, many later suffered unusual sequelae including atypical Parkinson's disease.[2]

Vaccines have been a medical breakthrough that has dramatically reduced death from infectious agents. When an infant is vaccinated, the purpose of the vaccination is to improve immunity to a particular disease. A vaccine typically contains an agent(s) that resembles a disease-causing microorganism, and it is often made from weakened or killed forms of the microbe or its toxins. The vaccine stimulates the body's adaptive (T_H2) immune system to identify the agent(s) as foreign, destroy it, and "recognize" it, so that the immune system can more easily recognize and destroy any of the microorganisms that it later encounters.[3]

Functions of the adaptive immune system (T_H2) in allergies include the following.

- Recognition of specific "non-self" antigens in the presence of "self," during the process of antigen presentation.
- Generations of responses that is tailored to maximally eliminate allergens.
- Development of immunological memory, in which each allergen is "remembered" by a signature IgE.

In summary, adaptive immunity may be thought of as an active army. This army provides us with the ability to recognize and remember the *Hevea*-allergens, and to mount stronger attacks each time the *Hevea*-allergens are encountered.

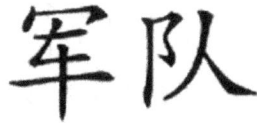

Army

- Invasion = *Hevea*-allergen contaminated vaccine
- Enemy = Foreign proteins
- Soldiers = IgE
- Theater of Operation = Human body
- Spies = *Hevea*-allergen structure homology
- Friendly Fire = IgE Cross-reactivity
- Out-of-Control Army = Atopy
- Casualties = Anaphylactic shock, Autoimmunity, Allergy-induced regressive autism

---

It is reasonable to assume that every protein component in a vaccine may be recognized as an enemy combatant. In this book, it will be shown that the allergens in *HDNR* (*Hevea*-allergens) can affect the incidence of atypical immunity. When *Hevea*-allergen sensitivity is acquired from vaccines that use *HDNR*, an atypical immunity response may induce atopy and affect the incidence of allergy-induced regressive autism.

Allergy-induced autism is an area of research wherein immune responses to certain environmental proteins, and foodstuff proteins, may affect the development and intensity of atypical behaviors within the autism spectrum.

The *Hevea*-allergens in natural latex are known to cause severe and pervasive immune responses. In children and adults, repeated exposure to such allergens has been shown to cause an increased incidence of sensitization, adverse allergic reactions, and even death through anaphylactic shock.

In the Nova Science book entitled "*Allergies and Autism,*" researchers describe how *HDNR* allergens may cause allergy-induced autism. The immune-response perspective describes how certain environmental proteins may affect neuro-cognitive development in children. Specifically, proteins inherent in natural latex are known to cause severe and pervasive immune responses. More specifically, the *Hevea brasiliensis* proteins in natural latex may trigger IgE mediated reaction antibodies and influence cross-reacting immune responses to other exogenous/endogenous proteins. Natural latex has seen a dramatic increase in usage over the last thirty years (e.g., health care industry, consumer products). The timing, frequency, intensity, and type of exposure to such proteins may influence the incidence, degree of atypicality, and prevalence of ASD. The researchers suggest that efforts should be directed at exploring how immune responses to such proteins affect lymphocyte sensitivity, enzyme regulation, and neural formation during prenatal/neonatal development.[4]

Furthermore, repeated exposure to the *Hevea*-allergens that are present in consumer products, including baby bottles, nipples, and pacifiers further intensifies atopy and allergy-induced regressive autism. More details on the hazards of infant products containing *Hevea*-allergens are discussed in Chapter 8 (Unhealthy Absorption).

When the body defends against pathogens, does it affect neural growth?

It has been shown that circulating neuron growth factor (NGF) levels are increased in humans with allergic diseases. The highest NGF values were found in patients with severe allergic asthma, a high degree of bronchial hyper-reactivity, and high total IgE and eosinophil cationic protein serum levels.[5]

Neurotrophin, including NGF and brain-derived neurotrophic factor (BDNF), are endogenous proteins critical for the survival and maintenance of neurons and lymphocyte expression. In fact, the 1986 Nobel Prize in Medicine was awarded to Stanley Cohen and Rita Levi-Montalcini for work showing that NGF is an extremely potent biological substance for the growth of sensory and sympathetic nerves.

The discovery of NGF in the beginning of the 1950s is a fascinating example of how a skilled observer can create a concept out of apparent chaos. Until this time, experimental neurobiologists did not understand how the development of the nervous system was regulated to result in the final complete innervations of the body. The investigation of NGF's role in the development of the nervous system, as well as later, in adult neural function, has been a lifelong dedication for Levi-Montalcini. Developmental biologist Levi-Montalcini, who in the beginning of 1950s moved from her homeland Italy to Viktor Hamburger's laboratory in St. Louis, USA, showed in 1952 that when tumors from mice were transplanted to chick embryos, they induced potent growth of the chick embryo nervous system, specifically sensory and sympathetic nerves. Because outgrowth did not require direct contact between the tumor and the chick embryo, Levi-Montalcini concluded that the tumor released a nerve-growth-promoting factor that had a selective action on certain types of nerves. Following this discovery, Levi-Montalcini turned to a more sensitive cell culture system in order to measure NGF activity in various extracts. NGF proved to be an extremely potent biological substance, with sensory or sympathetic nerve cells reacting within thirty seconds to the addition of minute quantities of NGF in herd studies. One-billionth part of a gram of NGF per ml of culture medium exerted a potent growth-promoting effect. A few minutes after the addition of NGF, nerve fibers began to grow out from the ganglion, which after a day's exposure to NGF resembled a sun surrounded by rays. This biological assay to detect NGF paved the way for the next step in this pathway of discovery and identification of the active nerve-growth-promoting substance. The recent finding of NGF in the brain has raised great expectation. An important pathway in the brain with acetylcholine as a transmitter substance seems to be sensitive to NGF.[6]

Nerve growth factor not only acts on nervous system development, but also has an important role in immune system physiology. Memory B-cells, lymphocytes that keep memory of an organism's encounter with a given chemical structure (antigen), produce and secrete NGF, bind it through cell surface receptors, and respond to its biologic message (autocrine circuit of production and response by the same cell). These memory B-cells remain alive for many years, or even throughout the life of the organism, at variance with the rest of the lymphoid cells, which have a much shorter life span. Beyond the activity of NGF in maintaining survival of memory B-cells, NGF might also influence their generation, positively acting on their precursors. The memory cell could originate from the ability of producing NGF, stochastically acquired by a progenitor otherwise destined to death by apoptosis (suicide), which would give rise to the autocrine loop-sustaining differentiation to the stage of mature memory cell, and then survival of the latter.

A study has shown that circulating NGF levels are increased in humans with allergic diseases. NGF serum levels were measured in forty-nine patients with asthma and/or rhino-conjunctivitis and/or urticaria-angioedema. Clinical and biochemical parameters, such as bronchial reactivity, total and specific serum IgE levels, and circulating eosinophil cationic protein levels were evaluated in relation to NGF values in asthma patients. NGF was significantly increased in the forty-two allergic (skin-test- or radio-allergosorbent-test-positive) subjects (49.7 +/- 28.8 pg/ml) versus the eighteen matched controls (3.8 +/- 1.7 pg/ml; P < 0.001). NGF levels in allergic patients with asthma, rhino-conjunctivitis, and urticaria-angioedema were 132.1 +/- 90.8, 17.6 +/- 6.1, and 7.6 +/- 1.8 pg/ml (P < 0.001, P < 0.002, and P < 0.05 versus controls), respectively. Patients with more than one allergic disease had higher NGF serum values than those with a single disease. When asthma patients were considered as a group, NGF serum values (87.6 +/- 59.8 pg/ml) were still significantly higher than those of control groups (P < 0.001), but allergic asthma patients had elevated NGF serum levels compared with non-allergic asthma patients (132.1 +/- 90.8 versus 4.9 +/- 2.9 pg/ml; P < 0.001). NGF serum levels correlate to total IgE serum values (rho = 0.43; P < 0.02). The highest NGF values were found in patients with severe allergic asthma, a high degree of bronchial hyper-reactivity, and high total IgE and eosinophil cationic protein serum levels. This study represents the first observation (that we know of) that NGF levels are increased in human allergic inflammatory diseases and asthma.[7]

Furthermore, increased levels of NGF have been shown to induce growth and differentiation of human B lymphocytes (B-cells). The principal functions of B-cells are to make antibodies against antigens, perform the role of antigen presenting cells, and eventually develop into memory B-cells after activation by antigen interaction. Thus, B-cells are an essential component of the adaptive immune system.[8]

Can the over-expression of NGF affect autism?

NGF over-expression has been linked to autism. In a study, investigators examined and compared archived neonatal blood samples from children born in four northern California counties from 1983 to 1985 who later developed autism, mental retardation, or cerebral palsy, or who developed normally. The investigators measured concentrations of several neural growth factors and found that the growth factors were significantly elevated in the neonatal blood of children who later developed autism or mental retardation, but not in the blood from children who developed cerebral palsy or blood from the normal controls.[9]

The Hevea-allergens are terroristic proteins. – Michael J. Dochniak

———

Notes

1. "Virus," Wikipedia, The free encyclopedia, http://en.wikipedia.org/wiki/Virus, accessed 1/11/11.
2. George Moore, "Influenza and Parkinson's Disease," *Public Health Reports,* 92, 1 (1977):79-80.
3. "Vaccine," Wikipedia, The free encyclopedia, http://en.wikipedia.org/wiki/Vaccine, accessed 1/11/11.
4. M.J. Dochniak, D.H. Dunn, *Allergies and Autism,* Allergies and Infectious Diseases Series (NY: Nova Science, 2010).
5. Sergio Bonini, Alessandro Lambiase, Stefano Bonini, et al., "Circulating Nerve Growth Factor Levels Are Increased in Humans with Allergic Diseases and Asthma, *PNAS* 93, 20 (1996):10955-10960.
6. "The Nobel Prize in Physiology or Medicine," Nobelforsamlingen Kardinska Institutet (1986), accessed 1/11/11, http://nobelprize.org/nobel_prizes/medicine/laureates/1986/press.html.

7. Bonini et al., "Circulating Nerve Growth."
8. U. Otten, P. Ehrhard, and R. Peck, "Nerve Growth Factor Induces Growth and Differentiation of Human B Lymphocytes, *Proc Natl Acad Sci* 86 (1989):10059-10063.
9. K.B. Nelson et al., "Neuropeptides and Neurotrophins in Neonatal Blood of Children with Autism or Mental Retardation." Annals of Neurology, May 2001, Vol. 49[5], 597-606.).

———

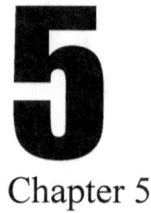

Chapter 5

Vaccination
Virus and bacteria to make benign
Brilliant vaccine, adjuvant supreme, immunity extreme
Antibodies to...
Discriminate, dominate, and terminate

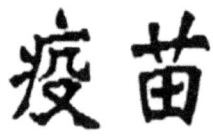

Vaccine

———

Vaccine Karma

Mans' survival is continually being challenged by invading armies of pathogens, including viruses and bacteria. Protection from these tiny but infinite pathogens, through forced immunity (i.e., vaccine), has allowed many of us to live longer and healthier lives. Vaccines are designed to be incapable of causing severe infection. A vaccine is a preparation of a weakened or killed pathogen, or a portion of the pathogen structure, that upon administration stimulates antibody production and immunity. For example, subunit vaccines use only a portion of the pathogen (e.g., the capsid proteins of the virus) to initiate forced immunity.

Vaccines make a qualitative difference in the lives of many people. As an example, before tetanus (lockjaw) immunization was available, the fear of tetanus infection lingered over every puncture wound or break in the skin. Some may recall the vigor with which every childhood scrape was scrubbed and doused with stinging antiseptics to prevent infections. Tetanus is now very rare in the United States, due to regular tetanus immunizations and boosters.

In 1952, polio paralyzed more than twenty-one thousand people. In 2002, there were no cases of polio in the United States, due to polio vaccinations.

Prior to 1985, Haemophilus Influenzas type-b (Hib) caused serious infections in twenty thousand children each year, including twelve thousand cases of meningitis. As a result of the Hib vaccination, there were only thirty-four cases of Hib disease in 2002.

In a cost-benefit analysis of Hib vaccination, researchers concluded that a nationwide Hib vaccination program should be started because the monetary benefits to society of such a program would exceed the costs to society.[1]

In the 1964-1965 rubella epidemics, there were 12.5 million cases of rubella. Of the twenty thousand infants born with congenital rubella syndrome, 11,600 were deaf, 3,580 were blind, and 1,800 were mentally retarded as a result of the infection. There were only nine cases of rubella in 2004 and only four cases of congenital rubella between 2001 and 2004.[2]

These examples show that herd vaccination is an effective means of reducing infectious disease. Herd immunity occurs when the vaccination of a portion of the population (or herd) provides protection to unprotected individuals. Herd immunity theory proposes that, in diseases passed from person to person, it is more difficult to maintain a chain of infection when large numbers of a population are immune. The spreading of a disease is reduced when a greater number of individuals have immunity to that disease.

Why waste another breath vilifying the anti-vaccination minority when steps can be taken to expand the pro-vaccination majority? – (Michael Willrich, Associate Professor of history at Brandeis University)

It is also becoming clear that there is risk associated with vaccinations. For example, researchers have shown that infection of human B-cells with rhinovirus or measles virus could lead to the initial steps of IgE class switching. Class switch recombination allows the body to produce antibodies with different effector functions, that is, a different means of dealing with the same antigen. The commonly used live attenuated measles mumps rubella (MMR) vaccine was selected for evaluation. Results showed that infection of a human IgM+ B-cell line with MMR resulted in the expression of germ line e transcript. In addition, infection of freshly prepared human peripheral blood lymphocytes with this vaccine resulted in the expression of mature IgE mRNA transcript. The data suggest that a potential side effect of vaccination with live attenuated viruses may be an increase in the expression of IgE.[3]

If vaccinations increase the expression of IgE, what type of allergies may be affected?

Research has shown that the odds of having a history of asthma were twice as great among vaccinated subjects compared to un-vaccinated subjects. Furthermore, the odds of having any allergy-related respiratory symptom was 63 percent greater among vaccinated subjects compared to unvaccinated subjects.[4]

Manufacturers of vaccines do encourage physicians to report suspected adverse events through the *Vaccine Adverse Event Reporting System*, which is sponsored by the CDC and FDA. If vaccine injury does occur, there is financial compensation to the severely disabled. For example, the U.S. Department of Health and Human Services has set up the National Vaccine Injury Compensation Program in 1988 to compensate individuals and families of individuals injured by covered childhood vaccines.[5] The program was established by the 1986 National Childhood Vaccine Injury Act (NCVIA), passed by the United States Congress in response to a threat to the vaccine supply due to a 1980s scare over the DPT vaccine.[6]

Can contaminated vaccines create a subgroup of autism?

———

Vaccine stopper of dry rubber, *Hevea-allergen* danger
Infant selected, then is injected, immunity affected
Antibodies to know, antibodies to grow
Antibodies live, antibodies give
Hevea-allergen contamination, body and mind to damage
Latex allergy offend, sympathetic neural networks over-extend
Allergy-induced regressive autism

———

The release of *Hevea*-allergens from the HDNR components of vaccine stoppers and prefilled syringes into aqueous pharmaceuticals may potentially induce latex sensitivity or an immediate natural-latex allergic reaction in atopic individuals.

Facts do not 'speak for themselves', they are read in the light of theory.
- Stephan Jay Gould (1941-2002)

Described below is a mechanism of how *Hevea*-allergen-contaminated vaccines may affect the incidence of allergy-induced regressive autism:

1. An atopic child is insulted with a vaccine contaminated with *Hevea*-allergens, inducing atypical activation of adaptive immunity.
2. The child's adaptive immune system develops memory B-cells that recognize the *Hevea*-allergens, thereby causing latex allergy.

3.   Latex allergy induces IgE cross-reactivity, further intensifying atopy (e.g., food allergies).
4.   Atopy affects neurological development through the over expression of NGF.

How do the *Hevea*-allergens affect atypical activation of adaptive immunity?

The incidence and prevalence of *Hevea*-allergen-specific memory B-cells play an important role in atopy and allergy-induced regressive autism. Memory B-cells make IgE specific to the *Hevea*- allergens. These B-cells can survive for long periods and, thus, impart a "memory" to the immune response.

It is speculated that *Hevea*-allergen-specific memory B-cells, and IgE cross-reactivity there from, play an important role in atopy and allergy-induced regressive autism.   In support, individuals with elevated levels of IgE (i.e., Job's syndrome) do not show a higher incidence of atopy or allergy-induced regressive autism. A study showed that patients with Hyper-IgE syndrome had reduced memory B-cells.[7] In summary, reduced memory B-cells can decrease the incidence and prevalence of allergen-specific IgE and cross-reactivity there from.

Why is it so very important to have *HDNR*-free vaccines?

Research has shown that natural-latex vial closures can release allergenic latex proteins into the tested solutions through direct contact during storage, and the release can occur in sufficient quantities to elicit positive intradermal skin reactions in some individuals with latex allergy. The researchers concluded that the data support a recommendation to eliminate natural latex from closures of pharmaceutical vials.[8] Furthermore, subjecting infants to even minutes quantities of such allergens could cause sensitization and latex allergy.

Fortunately, the U.S. government continues to address this issue. For example, in 2010 the FDA warned of natural-latex reactions from flu vaccines. Specifically, concerns about natural-latex labeling have led to FDA-mandated warnings for several prominent flu vaccines. More specifically, the flu vaccines manufactured by GlaxoSmithKline, Sanofi Pasteur, and Novartis Vaccines and Diagnostics, are alleged to contain natural-latex tips, which may cause allergic reactions, the American Academy of Family Physicians reports. GlaxoSmithKline said that that fewer flu vaccine doses would be available as a result, while Sanofi Pasteur said that shipments would be delayed by two to three weeks as a result of the new warnings. Novartis Vaccines and Diagnostics also informed customers that its syringe tips might contain natural latex.[9]

A Sanofi Pasteur notice describing the labeling change is as follows, "In mid-July, the FDA made us aware that after completing a review of the 'latex-free' claim made by the supplier of multiple influenza vaccines' syringe tip caps, it concluded there was insufficient documentation to support that claim. As a result, the Prescribing Information (PI) for Fluzone vaccine has been revised and now states that the tip caps 'may contain natural latex.' This affects all injectable influenza vaccine manufacturers who use the syringe cap supplied by Helvoet Pharma. This unexpected and relatively late change by the FDA is beyond our control, and affected the labeling and packaging for all presentations of Fluzone vaccine, resulting in an impact to our original shipping timelines." [10]

Unfortunately, oral vaccines are another vaccination delivery-system that may contain natural latex. An example includes the rotavirus-vaccine Rotarix®, manufactured by GlaxoSmithKline Biologicals. The tip cap and the rubber plunger of the oral applicator contain dry natural rubber. It has been recommended that infants with a severe (anaphylactic) allergy to natural latex should not be given Rotarix®.

In Chapter 10 (Safety First), vaccine safety procedures and blood tests are suggested, which may be used to reduce or eliminate the incidence of atopy and allergy-induced regressive autism in children.

Atopic infant be protected
Inspection before injection

In summary, the integrity of the immune system is required for 'typical' neurological development. *Hevea*-allergen contamination from the *HDNR* component of vaccines continues to put the mental health of children at risk. It is time to eliminate *HDNR* in all medical applications!

The solution to adult problems tomorrow depends on large measure upon how our children grow up today. – Margaret Mead (American Anthropologist)

————

Notes

1. G.M. Ginsberg et al., Cost Benefit Analysis of Haemophilus Influenza Type B Vaccination Programme in Israel, *J Epidemiology Community Health* 47 (1993): 485-490.
1. R.F. Edlich et al., "Update on the National Vaccine Injury Compensation Program." *Journal of Emergency Medicine* 33, 2 (2007):199-211.
2. Imani Farhad et al., "Infection of Human B Lymphocytes with MMR Vaccine Induces IgE Class Switching," *J. Clinical Immunology* 100, 3 (2001):355-361.
3. Eric L. Herwitz et al., "Effects of Diphtheria-Tetanus-Pertussis or Tetanus Vaccination on Allergies and Allergy-related Respiratory Symptoms among Children and Adolescents in the United States," *Journal of Manipulative and Physiological Therapeutics*, 23, 2 (2000):81-90.
4. W. Atkinson et al., eds., *Epidemiology and Prevention of Vaccine-Preventable Diseases* (The

Pink Book), 6th ed. (Atlanta: Centers for Disease Control and Prevention, 2000).

5.   "Vaccine Court," Wikipedia, The free Encyclopedia, http://en.wikipedia.org/wiki/ Vaccine_court, accessed 1/11/11.

6.   C. Speckmann et al., "Reduced Memory B cells in Patients with Hyper IgE Syndrome," *Clinical Immunology* 129, 3 (2008): 448-454.

7.   M.N. Primeau et al., "Natural Rubber Pharmaceutical Vial Closures Release Latex Allergens That Produce Skin Reactions," *J. Allergy Clin. Immunol.* 107, 6 (2001):958-62.

8.   Malik Wilson, "FDA Warns of Latex Reactions from Flu Vaccines," August 26, 2010, Vaccine DailyNews. com, http://vaccinenewsdaily.com/news/214867-fda-warns-of-latex-reactions-from-flu-vaccines, accessed 1/11/11.

9.   Sanofi Pasteur, "Latex Labeling Change Notice," August 2010, http://www.doh.state.fl.us/disease_ctrl/immune/files/Fluzone.pdf, accessed 1/11/11.

———

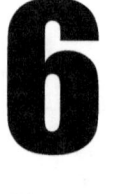

Chapter 6

Immunologic adjuvants antigen juiced
Aluminum hydroxide umpteen boosts
Latex contamination
Tainted vaccine
Aluminum to find aluminum to bind
Forced immunity
Misaligned

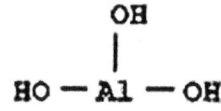

Aluminum hydroxide

———

Adjuvants Seduce

Aluminum hydroxide is the only adjuvant approved for routine use in humans and tends to skew immunity toward adaptive immunity. An adjuvant is defined as any substance that acts to accelerate, prolong, or enhance antigen-specific immune responses when used in combination with specific vaccine antigens.

It is generally understood that an adjuvant in vaccines enhances both innate (T_H1) and adaptive (T_H2) immunity. Research indicates that adjuvants exert their immune-enhancing effects as follows.

- Adjuvants help in the translocation of antigens to the lymph nodes where they can be recognized by T-cells. This will ultimately lead to greater T-cell activity resulting in a heightened clearance of pathogen throughout the organism.
- Adjuvants provide physical protection to antigens, which grants the antigen a prolonged delivery. This means that the organism will be exposed to the antigen for a longer duration, making the immune system more robust as it makes use of the additional time by up regulating the production of B-cells and T-cells needed for greater immunological memory in the adaptive immune response.
- Adjuvants help to increase the capacity to cause local reactions at the injection site (during vaccination), inducing greater release of danger signals by chemokine-releasing cells such as helper T-cells and mast cells.
- Adjuvants induce the release of inflammatory cytokines, which help recruit B-cells and T-cells and increase transcriptional events, leading to a net increase of immune cells.[1]

Does an aluminum-hydroxide □ *Hevea*-allergen complex induce regressive autism?

We've seen that *HDNR* continues to be associated with vaccine delivery system components including vial stoppers, syringe stoppers, needle shields, and syringe tip caps. When aluminum hydroxide is present in a vaccine solution, *Hevea*-allergen contamination could form an aluminum hydroxide □ *Hevea*-allergen complex that more readily causes latex allergy. The following mechanism is proposed.

1. A vaccine contains the immunologic adjuvant aluminum hydroxide.

2. Inclusive in the vaccine is *HDNR*, which is present in the vaccine cap and/or syringe plunger tip.

3. *Hevea*-allergens leach from the *HDNR* into the aqueous vaccine to form an aluminum hydroxide □ *Hevea*-allergen complex:

H3N+CHRCOO- + (OH) Al(OH)-3 to H2NCHRCOOAl (OH)-3 + H2O

(Hevea-allergen) (Aluminum hydroxide) (Complex) (Water)

2H3N+CHRCOO- + (OH)Al(OH)-3 to (H2NCHRCOO) 2Al(OH) + 2H2O

3H3N+CHRCOO- + (OH)Al(OH)-3 to (H2NCHRCOO) 3Al + 3H2O

4. An infant is insulted with the aluminum hydroxide □ *Hevea*-allergen complex through vaccination;

Vaccine solution

+

H2NCHRCOOAl(OH)-3

2. The aluminum hydroxide □ *Hevea*-allergen complex triggers a T_H2 immune response that can induce latex allergy and atopy.

3. Atypical atopy induces the over-expression of NGF, affecting atypical neurological development and regressive autism.

It is well documented that many infant vaccines solutions contain aluminum hydroxide. Examples of children vaccines that have contained aluminum hydroxide include DTaP (for Diphtheria, Tetanus, and Pertussis), DTaP-Hepatitis B-Polio combination, DTaP-HIB-Polio combination, Hepatitis A, Hepatitis B, Haemophilus influenzae B(HIB), Human Papilloma Virus (HPV), and Pneumococcal vaccines.[2] Examples of vaccines that contain *HDNR* include DTap (for Diphtheria, Tetanus, and Pertussis), DTaP-Hepatitis B-Poliocombination, DTaP-HIB-Polio combination, Hepatitis A, Hepatitis B, Haemophilus influenzae B(HIB), Human Papilloma Virus (HPV), and Pneumococcal vaccines.[3]

Compounding the problem, the use of aluminum hydroxide has increased in some vaccines. For example, from 1999 to 2002 several mercury-laced vaccines were phased out of the recommended immunization schedule.

They were replaced with low-mercury, or "Thimerosal-free" vaccines. However, during this "phase-out," four doses of a new vaccine containing high aluminum content were added to the childhood immunization schedule (for pneumococcal disease). Two doses of another aluminum-containing vaccine (for Hib) were added in 2005—a 20 percent increase in aluminum content since the mercury phase-out. While aluminum by itself is not toxic in trace amounts, the amount in vaccines can be as high as 0.5 percent.

Furthermore, it is known that aluminum hydroxide effectively binds to the *Hevea* allergens. For example, U.S. Patent 7,056,970 (Honeycutt) discloses a method for reducing allergenicity of natural latex. The natural latex, prior to its vulcanization, is admixed with aluminum hydroxide to denature the antigenic protein, thus reducing the total protein level considerably. Most of the aluminum-hydroxide □ *Hevea*-allergen complex is separated from the aqueous natural-latex dispersion by filtration or centrifugation to provide an ultra-low-protein *Hevea brasiliensis* natural-rubber latex product.[4]

How do we know that an aluminum-hydroxide □ *Hevea*-allergen complex may be harmful to humans?

In animal studies, mice have been intraperitoneal injected with *Hevea*-allergens that are adsorbed onto aluminum hydroxide gel, inducing natural-latex allergy.[5]

Therefore, as a safety precaution companies that deproteinize natural latex using aluminum hydroxide need to determine if an undesirable quantity of aluminum-hydroxide □ *Hevea*-allergen remains in the final product.

Unfortunately, medical science has not determined what level of the *Hevea*-allergens is considered safe. For example, it has been suggested that a *Hevea*-allergen concentration less than 50 µg/gram (1 µg = 0.000,001 grams) of water-soluble *Hevea*-allergens will limit sensitization in most individuals. However, some immune-sensitive individuals could react if exposed to one part per billion (i.e., 1 part in 10^9 parts).[6] An aluminum-hydroxide ☐ Hevea-allergen complex could lower the threshold of sensitization even further.

How does aluminum hydroxide increase immunity?

Studies have shown that aluminum hydroxide affects dendritic cell and macrophage activity. Dendritic cells (DCs) are immune cells that process antigens and present them on the surface to other cells of the immune system, thus functioning as antigen-presenting cells. Once activated, they migrate to the lymphoid node, where they interact with T-cells and B-cells to initiate and shape the adaptive immune response. A study evaluated the role of aluminum-hydroxide adjuvant in antigen internalization by dendritic cells *in vitro*. The researchers concluded that antigen internalization by dendritic cells was enhanced when the antigen remained adsorbed to the aluminum-containing adjuvant following administration.[7]

Furthermore, macrophage cells play an important role in forced immunity. Macrophages are phagocytes that engulf pathogens, digest pathogens, and stimulate lymphocytes and other immune cells to respond to the pathogens. A study investigated the *in vitro* effect of aluminum hydroxide adjuvant on isolated macrophages. Researchers disclosed that aluminum hydroxide-loaded macrophages exhibited phenotypical and functional modifications, as they expressed the classical markers of myeloid dendritic cells and displayed potent ability to induce MHC-II-restricted antigen-specific memory responses, but kept macrophage morphology. This suggests a key role of macrophages in the reaction to aluminum hydroxide adjuvant vaccines, and these mature antigen-presenting macrophages may, therefore, be of particular importance in the establishment of memory responses and in vaccination mechanisms leading to long-lasting protection.[8]

In other immunological twists and turns, it has been shown that aluminum hydroxide may be a useful adjuvant for inclusion in allergen immunotherapy vaccines. Allergen immunotherapy is a form of immunotherapy for allergic disorders in which the patient is vaccinated with increasingly larger doses of an allergen (substances to which they are allergic) with the aim of inducing immunologic tolerance. A study evaluated aluminum hydroxide effects on secondary allergic responses in humans. Researchers showed that aluminum hydroxide down-regulates allergen-driven T_H2 cytokine responses while T_H1 cytokines are unaffected. Peripheral blood mononuclear cells from atopic donors cultured with an allergen and aluminum hydroxide showed a significant decrease in both Interleukin-5 (IL-5) and IL-13 production compared with the allergen alone.[9]

It is clear that aluminum hydroxide has played a major role in the efficacy of vaccines. Unfortunately, it is also understood that vaccines that use *HDNR* may contaminate the vaccine with *Hevea*-allergens and form a dangerous aluminum-hydroxide □ *Hevea*-allergen complex. It is this complex that may be a catalyst for the development of atopy and allergy-induced regressive autism.

Mankind beware, aluminum hydroxide and Hevea-allergens are a troubling combination – Michael J. Dochniak

———

Notes

1. V. Schijns, "Immunological Concepts of Vaccine Adjuvant Activity," *Curr. Opin. Immunol.* 12, 4 (2000):456-63.
2. MOTHERING, No. 146, January-February 2008, pp. 46-53.
3. Johns Hopkins Bloomberg School of Public Health, Institute for Vaccine Safety, http://www.vaccinesafety.edu/components-Allergens.htm, accessed 1/11/11.

4. U.S. Patent 7,056,970 (Honeycutt),"Decreasing allergenicity of natural rubber latex prior to vulcanization," June 6 (2006).

5. Charles L. Hardy et al., "Characterization of a Mouse Model of Allergy to a Major Occupational Latex Glove allergen Hev-b 5," *American Journal of Respiratory and Critical Care Medicine* 167 (2003):1393-1399.

6. Blood Borne Pathogens Self-Study Module-Preventing Skin and Mucocutaneous Exposures, http://www.co.dare.nc.us/depts/EMS/Bloodborne/page24.htm, accessed 1/11/11.

7. G.L. Morefield et al., "Role of Aluminum-containing Adjuvants in Antigen Internalization by Dendritic Cells In Vitro," *Vaccine* 23, 13 (2005):1588-95.

8. A.C. Rimaniol et al., "Aluminum Hydroxide Adjuvant Induces Macrophage Differentiation towards a Specialized Antigen-presenting Cell Type," *Vaccine*, 22, 23-24 (2004):3127-35.

9. L.K. Wilcock et al., "Aluminum Hydroxide Down-Regulates T Helper 2 Responses by Allergen-stimulated Human Peripheral Blood Mononuclear Cells," *Clinical & Experimental Allergy*, 34, 9, (2004): 1373-1378.

7

Chapter 7

Androgens produce what regressive autism will induce
Sex hormones and immunity
No impunity
Testosterone profound
Antigens abound, antibodies around
If atopy assists then degranulation persists
Neurotrophin expression may bring about regression
NGF flows and neurons
Grow…and grow…and
grow…and grow…
and grow
Over-connectivity out of control
Androgens produce what atopy will induce
Regressive behaviors to grow
Regressive autism to know
Sex hormones and immunity
No impunity

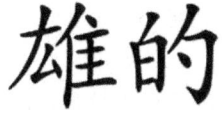

Gender

———

Gender Difference

Males are four times (4x) more likely to develop an ASD, compared to females.

Does the expression of testosterone shift immunity toward T_H2, increasing allergy-induced regressive autism in males?

A study has suggested that clear sex differences exist in atopy, with a preponderance of atopy in boys before puberty.[1]

Early infancy androgen effects are the least understood. In the first weeks of life for male infants, testosterone levels rise. The levels remain in a pubertal range for a few months, but usually reach the barely detectable levels of childhood by four to six months of age. The function of this rise in humans is unknown. It has been speculated that "brain masculinization" is occurring, because no significant changes have been identified in other parts of the body.[2]

Furthermore, researchers have shown that dissimilar immunity may exist in males and females. Specifically, cytokines may play an essential role, especially the cytokines released by T helper (T_H) lymphocytes. These cells respond to an immune challenge in one of two ways: T_H1 lymphocytes secrete interleukin-2 (IL-2), interferon-g (IFN-g), and lymphotoxin, establishing a pro-inflammatory environment, whereas T_H2 lymphocytes secrete IL-4, IL-5, IL-6, IL-10, and transforming growth factor-b (TGF-b), which promote antibody production. Both sets of lymphocytes exert cross-regulatory influences on each other. Research has established that females are more likely to develop a T_H1 response after challenge with an infectious agent or antigen, except during pregnancy when a T_H2 environment prevails.[3]

In continuation, research suggests that there may be a link between ASD and testosterone levels in the womb as the fetus develops. For example, research from Cambridge

University has shown that babies who produce high levels of testosterone while they are still in the womb have a higher chance of showing ASD traits later on.[4]

Described below is a mechanism of how vaccine-insult and elevated levels of testosterone may affect the incidence of allergy-induced regressive autism.

1. A child having an over-expression of testosterone is vaccinated, shifting immunity further towards T_H2.
2. Increased T_H2 lymphocytes secrete IL-4, IL-5, IL-6,and IL-10 further inducing atypical T_H2 antibody production.
3. Atypical expression T_H2 immune-cells induce atopy when sensitized to the *Hevea*-allergens.
4. Atopy can affect neurological development through the over-expression of NGF, resulting in allergy-induced regressive autism.

What do animal studies indicate about hormones and immunity?

Research on the differences in concentration of endogenous proteins in sex organs of BALB/c mice has shown that levels of NGF and IgE were consistently higher in organs of male mice in comparison to their female siblings.[5]

Females are four times (4x) less likely to develop an ASD, compared to males.

Does the expression of estrogen shift immunity toward T_H1 after vaccination, reducing allergy-induced regressive autism in females?

The three major naturally occurring estrogens are estriol, estradiol, and estrone. Estradiol is the predominant form in females.

The expression of certain cytokines in females may underlie sex differences in immunity, compared to males. For example, cytokines play an essential role in immunity; especially the cytokines released by T-helper (T_H) lymphocytes. Females are more likely to develop a T_H1 response after challenge with an infectious agent or antigen. T_H-lymphocytes secrete interleukin-2 (IL-2), interferon-g (IFN-g), and lymph toxin, establishing a pro-inflammatory environment.[6] Therefore, the incidence and atypicality of regressive autism is decreased in females because estrogen helps to maintain T_H1 immunity.

It is possible that *Hevea*-allergen contamination in vaccines, and other routes of such allergen exposure, can induce atypical T_H2 immunity in both genders, affecting the incidence of atopy and allergy-induced regressive autism.[7] All children need to be protected from the *Hevea*-allergens, before and after vaccinations.

If the over-expression of testosterone affects the etiology of atopy and allergy-induced regressive autism, males having elevated levels of testosterone, and T_H2 immune-cells, need to be exempt from herd vaccination programs.

Herd immunity, is it fair?

Is it unity?

If hormones were the same, the prevalence of autism based on gender would not be to blame. – Michael J. Dochniak

———

Notes

1. M Osman, "Therapeutic Implications of Sex Differences in Asthma and Atopy," *Disease of Childhood* 88, (2003):587-590.
2. "Testosterone," Wikipedia – The free encyclopedia, http://en.wikipedia.org/wiki/Testosterone, accessed 1/11/11.
3. Catherine C. Whitacre et al., "A Gender Gap in Autoimmunity," *Science* 283, 5406 (1999):1277-1278.

4.   Autism News, "Autism and Testosterone Levels in the Womb Possible Link," 2004, http://windowsupdatecenter.com/?id=198760218, accessed 1/11/11.
5.   Binie V. Lipps, "Age and Sex-related Difference in Levels of Nerve Growth Factor in Organs of BALB/c mice," *Journal of Natural Toxins* 11 (2002):387-391.
6.   Catherine C. Whitacre et al., "A Gender Gap in Autoimmunity," *Science* 283, 5406 (1999):1277-1278.
7.   "Latex Allergy," Emergency Nurses Association White Paper, http://www.ena.org/SiteCollectionDocuments/Position%20Statements/Latex_Allergy_-_ENA_White_Paper.pdf, accessed 1/11/11.

———

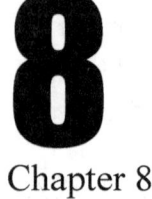

Chapter 8

Natural latex pacifier oh-so green, but are you really all that clean?
Soothing pacifier - lips to place, but are you really all that safe?
Suck, bite, and chew
Latex allergies may impair
Harmful proteins always there
Natural latex pacifier oh-so green
You're not healthy
You're not clean

Pacifier

———

Unhealthy Absorption

While the causes of ASD are complex and puzzling, a consensus is emerging that environmental triggers and atypical immunity likely play important roles. Government statistics suggest the prevalence rate of autism is increasing annually. According to the CDC, in the year 2006, the autism diagnosis rate was one in every 110 children; in 2009, it increased to one in every one hundred children.[1]

In the previous Chapters, we've seen how vaccinations can shift infant immunity towards T_H2 (i.e., allergies). Therefore, allergen exposure after vaccinations could dramatically affect an infant's sensitivity.

Are infants exposed to the *Hevea*-allergens after vaccination?

After vaccinations, infants are often exposed to products formed from *HDNR*, including baby bottle nipples, pacifiers, teething articles, medical devices, and medical packaging. In a research paper published in the journal *Medical Hypotheses*, it was disclosed that babies born in delivery rooms of hospitals are exposed to latex through skin and mucous membrane contact with pre-powdered latex gloves worn by midwives and doctors, and through the inhalation of latex-bound starch powder in the air of the delivery room. The paper examines the hypothesis that these babies are at risk for latex sensitization, and that part of the sharp increase of childhood asthma, eczema, and anaphylaxis in the past thirty to forty years may be linked to this exposure. These possibilities seem hitherto unsuspected. In over seven hundred papers on latex allergy, no mention of neonatal exposure to latex has been found. Even obstetric papers discussing the risks for an atopic mother (atopy - a tendency to develop allergies) do not seem to anticipate any risk for the baby, who might also be atopic. Latex allergy is primarily regarded as an occupational hazard. The *Medical Hypotheses* paper suggests that it is a hazard for every baby handled by latex gloves at birth.[2]

How is the government responding to medical products formed from *HDNR*?

The FDA has issued a guidance document entitled, "User Labeling for Devices That Contain Natural latex (21 CFR

801.437); Small Entity Compliance Guide." The document is intended to help manufacturers of medical products that contain NRL, the majority of whom are small businesses. The guidance addresses specific federal regulations for labeling medical products that contain NRL. In the document, the FDA refers to an increase in the number of deaths reported to the agency that are associated with an apparent sensitivity to natural-latex proteins contained in medical devices. Scientific studies and case reports have documented sensitivity to natural-latex proteins found in a wide range of medical devices. In order to protect the public health and minimize the risks associated with the use of natural-latex protein, the FDA has developed a labeling regulation that provides important information to individuals who are sensitive to natural-latex proteins. The final rule identifies specific labeling statements for use on medical devices and device packaging when they contain natural latex that contacts humans. The labeling requirements are as follows.

- Labeling of medical devices containing natural rubber latex that contacts humans should state: *Caution: This Product Contains Natural Rubber Latex Which May Cause Allergic Reactions.*
- Labeling of medical devices containing dry natural rubber latex that contacts humans should state: *This Product Contains Dry Natural rubber latex.*
- Labeling of medical devices containing natural rubber latex in their packaging that contacts humans should state: *Caution: The Packaging of This Product Contains Natural Rubber Latex Which May Cause Allergic Reactions.*
- Labeling of medical devices containing dry natural rubber latex in their packaging that contacts humans should state: *The Packaging of This Product Contains Dry Natural Rubber latex.*
- The claim of hypo-allergenicity should be removed from the labeling of medical devices and medical packaging that contains *HDNR.*

Taking post-vaccination *Hevea*-allergen exposure a step further, it is potentially hazardous for infants to mouth products made from HDNR including bottle nipples, pacifiers, teething rings, and toys. In infants wherein the T_H2 function predominates (i.e., atopy), *Hevea*-allergen sensitivity could have an unbalanced effect on the T_H1/T_H2 immune system, causing much harm.

Correlation is not causation but it sure is a hint. – Edward Tufte (American Statistician)

Described below is a proposed mechanism of how sublingual absorption of the *Hevea*-allergens may affect the incidence of allergy-induced regressive autism.

1. The atopic infant is subjected to vaccination, triggering two immunological branches; a cell-mediated immune response (T_H1) and a humoral immune response (T_H2).
2. An atopic infant has, or acquires, *Hevea*-allergen sensitivity increasing T_H2 immunity (e.g., mouthing natural-latex products including baby bottle nipples, pacifiers, teething rings)
3. A comorbid factor such as the under-expression of the anti-inflammatory cytokine interleukin-10 may lead to increased T_H2 immunity.
4. The increased T_H2 immunity may induce regressive autism through NGF over-expression.

Sublingual absorption allows some *Hevea*-allergens to pass directly into the blood stream, further intensifying an adaptive immune response. Sublingual absorption is different from gastrointestinal tract absorption in that materials absorb directly into the circulatory system under the tongue do not pass to the liver and then travel out into systemic circulation. In sublingual adsorption, a chemical enters the mouth and contacts the mucous membrane or buccal mucosa. It then diffuses into the epithelium beneath the tongue. This region contains a high density of blood vessels, and as a result, through osmosis, the chemical quickly enters the blood stream at the sublingual artery. Thereafter, the chemical may be carried by blood flow to the connected lingual artery, which may take up the chemical and translate it to its source: the carotid artery, which is connected directly to the brain.

In Chapter 6 (Adjuvants Seduce), we discussed why aluminum hydroxide and *Hevea*-allergens are such a troubling combination. In continuation, the aluminum hydroxide also present in many baby formulas could be a troubling material when associated with the *Hevea*-allergens. For example, baby formulas often contain aluminum hydroxide as an additive (e.g., the concentration in infant formula is 0.225 mg/L and the concentration in soy-based formula is 0.46 to 0.93 mg/L).[3] The *Hevea*-allergens in natural-latex nipples can bind to the aluminum hydroxide present in the baby formula and form an aluminum-hydroxide ☐ *Hevea*-allergen complex having increased allergenicity.

Can an infant's life be threatened by sucking on natural-latex nipples and pacifiers?

The *Hevea*-allergens can leach from the natural-latex products and be absorbed under the tongue. If the infant has natural-latex sensitivity, an adverse immune response is possible. In support, latex allergy has been known to cause anaphylactic shock during sublingual immunotherapy.[4]

Taking a peak at endogenous proteins, a child's cytokine expression also affects T_H2 immunity. For example, it is known that the anti-inflammatory cytokine IL-10 displays a potent ability to suppress the antigen presentation capacity of antigen-presenting cells, thus counteracting excessive immunity in the human body. The under-expression of IL-10, which is often present in children with ASD, may affect the incidence of hyper-adaptive immunity and allergy-induced autism. A study has shown that children with ASD have increased activation of both T_H2 and T_H1 arms of the adaptive immune response, with T_H2 predominance, and without the compensatory increase in the regulatory cytokine IL-10.[5]

In other studies, it has been shown that children with autism have distinctly different immune system reactions based on cytokine expression. Specifically, researchers have shown that cytokine responses elicited by the T-cell, B-cell, and macrophage cell populations following their activation differs markedly in children with autism compared to age-matched children in the general population.[6]

Allergy-induced autism research continues to explored how certain proteins induce hyper- adaptive-immunity, thereby affecting regressive autism. As we've seen, allergies can increase the expression of neurotrophin, including NGF, affects neural growth and synaptic pruning.[7,8,9] Researchers have also revealed that the timing, frequency, intensity, and type of exposure to the *Hevea*-allergens can induce hyper-adaptive immunity, affecting the incidence and degree of atypicality of autistic behaviors.[10]

Furthermore, in a research paper entitled, "Allergic manifestations in autistic children: Relations to disease severity," researchers concluded that allergy may play a role in the pathogenesis of autism wherein allergic immune responses to some proteins (dietary protein and latex protein) may induce the production of brain auto-antibodies, which are found in many autistic children.[11]

HDNR continues to adversely affect health and safety. Through research, it will be shown that exposure to *HDNR* can induce allergy-induced regressive autism. For example, in a study from Peking University (China) researchers hypothesized that immune reactions triggered by close contact with natural latex might influence the functions of B-lymphocytes by altering expression of certain proteins identified in their experiments, thus contributing to the occurrence of autism.[12]

In a different immunological pathway, absorption of the *Hevea*-allergens under the tongue has been tested in immunotherapy. For some individuals, sublingual immunotherapy (SLIT) can be used to reduce allergy symptoms. A general criteria for selecting patients for SLIT include: the individual has a mild to moderate IgE-mediated disease, clinically relevant allergens are available, the individual has exhausted pharmacological and non-pharmacological therapeutic options, and the individual has adverse side-effects to allergy medication.[13] Sublingual immunotherapy has a low success rate in adults and is not recommended for infants.

Because natural-latex is a commodity material that has played a significant role in industrial societies, alternatives have been explored. For example, the chemical industry is aware of the latex allergy problem and has produced synthetic alternatives. For example, there is a synthetic rubber product based on polyisoprene (i.e., polymer in HDNR) that does not contain allergenic proteins. Goodyear Chemical makes cis 1,4 polyisoprene (NATSYN® 2200/2210), which can be used where natural latex is traditionally used, including baby bottle nipples and healthcare items.[14]

In summary, hospitals ban HDNR-based nipples and pacifiers in their facilities, parents should also keep them out of their baby's mouth.

All truth passes through three stages. First, it is ridiculed. Second, it is violently opposed. Third, it is accepted as being self-evident. – Arthur Schopenhauer (1788-1860)

———

Notes

1. Centers for Disease Control and Prevention, http://www.cdc.gov/ncbddd/features/counting-autism.html, accessed 1/11/11.
2. J. Worth, "Neonatal sensitization to latex" *Journal of Medical Hypotheses* 54, 5 (2000):729-33.
3. The Children's Hospital of Philadelphia, Vaccine Education Center,

http://www.chop.edu/service/vaccine-education-center/hot-topics/aluminum.html, accessed 1/11/11.

4. A. Antico et al., "Anaphylaxis by Latex Sublingual Immunotherapy," *Allergy* 61, 10 (2006):1236-1237.

5. C.A. Molloy et al., "Elevated Cytokine Levels in Children with Autism Spectrum Disorder, *J. Neuroimmunol* 172, 1-2 (2006):198-205.

6. UCDAVIS Health System, "Children with autism have distinctly different immune system reactions compared to typical children," May 5, 2005, http://www.ucdmc.ucdavis.edu/newsroom/releases/archives/mind/2005/immune_sys5-2005.html, accessed 1/11/11.

7. Sergio Bonini et al., "Circulating Nerve Growth Factor Levels Are Increased in Humans with Allergic Diseases and Asthma," *PNAS.* 93, 20 (1996): 10955-10960.

8. U. Otten, P. Ehrhard, and R. Peck, "Nerve Growth Factor Induces Growth and Differentiation of Human B Lymphocytes *Proc Natl Acad Sci USA* 86 (1989):10059-10063.

9. UniSci, "NGF Proteins Present at Birth Linked to Later Autism," http://www.unisci.com/stories/20012/0426011.html, accessed 1/11/11.

10. M.J. Dochniak, D.H. Dunn, Allergies *and Autism*, Allergies and Infectious Disease Series (NY: Nova Science Publisher, 2010).

11. Gehan A. Mostafa et al., "Allergic Manifestations in Autistic Children: Relation to Disease Severity, *J. Pediatr. Neurol.* 6, 2 (2008):115-123.

12. C. Shen et al., "A Proteomic Investigation of B Lymphocytes in an Autistic Family: A Pilot Study of Exposure to Natural Rubber Latex (NRL) May Lead to Autism, *J. Mol. Neurosci.* (2010).

13. World Allergy Organization, "Sub-Lingual Immunotherapy," *WAO Journal* (2009): 233-281,

http://www.worldallergy.org/publications/slit-wao-pp_final.pdf, accessed 1/11/11.

14. Goodyear Chemical, Product Data Sheet, NATSYN® 2200/2210, http://www.americasinternational.com/product_sheets/Goodyear/PDS/Natsyn_2200_&_2210.pdf, accessed 1/11/11.

———

9

Chapter 9

Newborn develops with promise and plan
Medical science, a physician that can
Injection for protection
Brings
A baby that cries while immunity flies
Reaction from Injection
Brings
Immunity gone crazy, atopy not lazy
Well-meant plans, misguided scams
Regressive autism, allergy induced
Something is clear; answers are near
Slowly or quickly, behaviors take hold
Expanding a spectrum
Let It Be Told

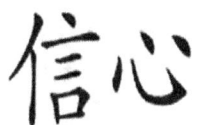

Confidence

———

Parent Confidence

The evidence is irrefutable, natural latex exposure is hazardous to adults and children. Studies show some 15 percent of healthcare workers are allergic to latex. The evidence of harm from the *Hevea*-allergens is well documented in the judicial system. As an example, a healthcare worker won £280,000 compensation from York Hospital after a seven-year fight over a potentially fatal allergy to everyday objects. Fiona Moore stated, "What they should have done is give me an environment in which I would be safe at work," she said. "I was told that wasn't cost-effective. I wasn't just a patient in the department, I worked there." [1, 2]

Furthermore, we've read in previous Chapters that HDNR has been widely used in the packaging and delivery system of childhood vaccines. Concerns about the use of HDNR in vaccines have been raised because of an increased awareness of the potential for adverse allergic-reactions to even low levels of the *Hevea*-allergens. HDNR is not banned for use in vaccines or prefilled syringes. But, US 21 Code of Federal Regulations (CFR) Part 8001.437 requires medical devices and drug packaging containing HDNR components to indicate on the product label that: "This product contains Dry Natural Rubber."

It is understood that reducing the protein levels in HDNR does not solve the problem in that the threshold of sensitivity to such proteins is unknown. Government agencies, emboldened to protect the health and safety of all Americans, including the CDC, FDA, National Vaccine Program Office (NVPO), and WHO have yet to set guidelines for safe exposure to the *Hevea*-allergens.

What is the *Hevea*-allergen standard for HDNR in vaccines?

There are protein standards for HDNR used in vaccine components and prefilled syringes. For example, HDNR components combined with prefilled syringes are subjected to initial qualification testing as part of the drug primary packaging. Specifically, biological testing for preclinical qualification must comply with the US Pharmacopeia (USP) 381, USP 88, Japanese Pharmacopeia (JP) 59, and ISO 10993 Parts 1, 5, 4, 10 and 11; cytotoxicity, acute systemic toxicity, intra-cutaneous reactivity (USP 88, ISO 10993-10), implantation test (USP 88, ISO 10993-6) sensitization by maximization test on guinea pigs (ISO 10993-10) after saline, and cotton seed oil extraction; and physicochemical tests according to European Pharmacopeia (EP) 3.2.9 and JP 59. The materials are tested and must pass satisfactory USP requirements for leachable and extractable materials. Notably, total protein contamination in aqueous extraction solution using the modified Lowry test must be below the detection limit of the measurement methods which is in parts per million.[3]

From a historical perspective, it has been shown that natural-latex in the medical-glove industry has done great harm. It is well known that health care workers and patients have experienced an increased number of sensitization from the use of powdered natural-latex gloves. The *Hevea*-allergens that have been shown to significantly affect the level of IgE primed cells are the water-soluble proteins (e.g., *Hev-b* 1-3). The allergen content of latex gloves has been shown to vary greatly and is due in part to protein leaching processing techniques. The International Rubber Research and Development Board have suggested that the *Hevea*-allergen problem appears to have been instigated by the appearance of some very poorly manufactured gloves and other natural-latex articles on the market. These were produced by entrepreneurs who were unaware of, or disregarded, normal natural-latex dipping plant management. At worst, they failed to maintain cleanliness on their dipping lines, thus permitting build-up of protein sediment in their dipping tanks. They also failed to ensure adequate leaching of their products, either through performing the operation too quickly, or through using contaminated water. This led to the marketing of some natural-latex products with very high protein levels. This in turn led to severe reactions in potentially sensitive individuals. There is also some evidence that the transfer of manufacture to natural-latex producing countries led to the use of fresh natural latex, which contains higher levels, and may make the seasonal and clonal variations in protein levels more pronounced in the products manufactured from them.[4]

Vaccines are a medical application where HDNR need not be used. It is very important to understand that, currently, the Hevea-allergens in HDNR cannot be completely removed. If even minute quantities of the Hevea-allergens leach into a vaccine they are then injected directly into the infant's body, which thereafter may produce serum antibodies inducing latex allergy.

Can Hevea brasiliensis genetic material leach into vaccines?

In speculation, genetic material in dry natural rubber, including plasmids and transposons, could leach into the vaccine's aqueous-solution. For example, according to the cellular origin hypothesis or vagrancy hypothesis, viruses can evolve from bits of DNA or RNA that "escape" from the genes. The escaped DNA or RNA could come from plasmids that are pieces of naked DNA or RNA that can move between cells or transposons, which are molecules of DNA that replicate and move around to different positions within the genes of the cell. Once called "jumping genes," transposons are examples of mobile genetic elements and could be the evolution of some viruses.

It is known that both DNA and RNA can be extracted from HDNR. For example, research has shown that expression of Hevein genes in natural latex has been detected.[5]

A study that evaluated particulate ribonucleoprotein components of HDNR showed that a significant proportion of the particulate RNA is found in the rubber layer.[6]

Messenger RNA (mRNA) is a molecule of RNA encoding a chemical "blueprint" for a protein product.

mRNA is transcribed from a DNA template, and carries coding information to the sites of protein synthesis.

In continuation, a study has shown that the latex allergen Hev-b 5 transcript is widely distributed after subcutaneous injection in BALB/c mice of their DNA vaccine. The researchers concluded that the rapid and widespread appearance of the Hev-b 5 transcript in the injected mice confirms that DNA is translocated from the injection site, transcribed, and expressed in immune and non-immune tissues after injection.[7]

It is further speculated that persistent infection from surviving viruses, inclusive with *Hevea* genetic material, could maintain *Hevea*-allergen (i.e., Hev-b protein) transcription and its associated memory B-cell population. In summary, viruses that produce *Hevea*-allergens will not allow the latex allergy to go into remission. In an effort to better understand vaccine induced atopy and multiple chemical sensitivity, research efforts need to explore the viability of the *vagrancy hypothesis* wherein genetic material from HDNR leaches into a vaccine comprising live or attenuated viruses. Scientists have shown that a viral vector can be used to make the *Hevea*-allergens. For example, the Hev-b 1 and Hev-b 3 allergens have been successfully produced using a chimeric tobacco mosaic virus.[8]

What other explanation can be used to show *Hevea*-allergen exposure must be reduced?

The collision theory of reaction rates teaches us that an important variable to covalent and non-covalent bond formation is the concentration of the reactants. Simply, the more reactants there are the more likely a bond will occur. This bond formation mechanism doesn't apply to the adaptive immune system wherein "few" allergens can induce an intense immune reaction. Within adaptive immunity, there is a chemical intelligence wherein immune cells recognize and attack even minute quantities of an allergen, sometimes producing anaphylactic shock. All individuals who have been previously exposed to the *Hevea*-allergens are at risk, in that re-exposure increases the probability of an adverse allergic response.

Is the *HDNR* in vaccines ethical?

The Advisory Committee on Immunization Practices (ACIP) and the American Academy of Family Physicians (AAFP) recommend the following: If a person reports a severe (anaphylactic) allergy to latex, vaccines supplied in vials or syringes that contain *HDNR* should not be administered, unless the benefit of vaccination outweighs the risk of an allergic reaction to the vaccine. For latex allergies other than anaphylactic allergies (e.g., a history of contact allergy to latex gloves), vaccines supplied in vials or syringes that contain dry natural rubber or dry NRL can be administered.[9]

It is generally understood that the first time a child is exposed to the *Hevea*-allergens large amounts of IgE are made if such proteins are recognized as foreign. These IgE then attach themselves to mast cells and basophiles to form IgE primed cells. Thereafter, re-exposure to the *Hevea*-allergens can cause latex allergy.

It is further understood that repeated exposure to even minute quantities of the *Hevea*-allergens from *HDNR* can increase the incidence of latex allergy.[10] It is the opinion of the authors that it is unethical to expose infants to the *Hevea*-allergens through multiple vaccinations, knowing such allergens could induce latex allergy and cross-react food allergies through repeated exposure.

Do parents trust the U.S. vaccination program?

In a survey by University of Michigan researchers, data showed that one in four U.S. parents believe some vaccines cause autism in healthy children. Lead author Dr. Gary Freed has stated, "Nine out of 10 parents believe that vaccination is a good way to prevent diseases for their children. Luckily their concerns don't outweigh their decision to get vaccines so their children can be protected from life-threatening illnesses." It has also been written that some doctors are taking a tough stand on parents who refuse to give their children vaccinations, asking such parents to find other doctors, and calling these parents "selfish." [11]

Allergic reactions to vaccines used to be of prime concern to pharmaceutical and vaccine makers. That changed after the passage of the Public Readiness and Emergency Preparedness Act of 2006 [PREP Act 42USC 247(d)-6d)] that, basically, exonerates vaccine makers of any damages from vaccines and/or vaccinations. A special vaccine court has been established, from which harmed individuals must seek permission to bring legal charges. Common tort law no longer applies to vaccine/ vaccination injury/damage.

It is important for parents of atopic children to know that there are no federal laws mandating vaccinations; laws are made at the state level. All fifty states permit medical exemptions; most allow exemptions based on religious beliefs, and over one-third of the states accept exemptions based on personal beliefs, including California.

Based on new scientific research that atopy may affect the etiology of allergy-induced regressive autism, it is recommended that all vaccines that have HDNR need to be discontinued. Furthermore, medical institutions need to be consistent and ban all uses of HDNR, independent of end-use and Hevea-allergen protein content.

Undetectable levels of Hevea-allergens, based on the current analytical procedures, do not mean that such vaccines are free of the Hevea-allergens. Therefore, repeated exposure through multiple vaccinations that use HDNR in its packaging or delivery system could cause an adverse allergic response in any child who has an aggressive immune system. The FDA, CDC, and NVPO can provide leadership, ensuring that all vaccine processes and components are free of HDNR. It's a contradiction when many medical institutions promote a latex-free environment but then allow the use of *HDNR* in vaccines. In Chapter 13 (The Change), the *Hevea*-allergens in flu vaccines are discussed further.

A survey by the National Foundation for Infectious Diseases (NFID) showed that 43 percent of Americans say they will not be getting the vaccine in fall, 2010. Another survey from the same group found a third of American mothers saying they have no plans to get a flu shot for their children.[12]

In 1988, the National Vaccine Injury Compensation Program (VICP) went into effect to compensate individuals and families of individuals who have been injured by covered childhood vaccinations. It uses a no-fault alternative dispute resolution system for resolving vaccine injury claims. Funding for claims of harm after 1988 comes from a patient fee of 75 ¢ per vaccination. To win an award, a claimant must show a causal connection; if medical records show a child has one of several listed adverse effects soon after vaccination; the assumption is that it was caused by the vaccine. The proof standard is the civil-law preponderance of the evidence, showing that causation was more likely than not.

The following is a summary of the code of federal regulations - 42 CFR 100.3 - Vaccine injury table.

- Anaphylactic shock
- Encephalopathy
- Reserved
- Seizure and convulsion
- Sequela
- Chronic arthritis
- Brachial neuritis
- Thrombocytopenic purpura
- Vaccine-strain measles viral infection
- Vaccine-strain polio viral infection[13]

If a parent feels that their child has been harmed by vaccines, it is important to know that under the *National Childhood Vaccine Injury Act*, a no-fault system, parents do not have to prove a vaccine caused their child's injury. The parent has to show that the child had an injury that could be caused by the vaccine. A specific example, my autistic child has (or had) allergies and the *HDNR* in vaccines (i.e., *Hevea*-allergen insult) affected his/her allergy-induced regressive autism.

If a drug is sold and stored in vials with a natural-latex stopper, no matter what precautions you take, latex allergens can contaminate that drug. – Robert Hamilton (Ph.D. professor of medicine at Johns Hopkins University)

———

Notes

1. Physorg.com, "Latex Banned at Johns Hopkins Hospital," January 18, 2008, http://www.physorg. com/news119886779.html, accessed 1/11/11.
2. Latex allergy Links, "Litigation," accessed 1/11/11, http://www.latexallergylinks.org/lit.html, The Press and http://www.yorkpress.co.uk/news/4777174. Fiona_Moore_wins___280k_compensation_from_ York_Hospital_over_latex_allergy/, accessed 1/11/11.
3. European Medical Device Technology (EMDT), "Dry Natural Rubber Components in Prefilled Syringes," http://www.emdt.co.uk/article/dry-natural-rubber-components-prefilled-syringes.
4. The International Rubber Research and Development Board, "Latex Protein Allergy: The Political Dimension," accessed 1/11/11, http://www.irrdb.com/irrdb/naturalrubber/latexallergy/causesoflatex.htm.
5. Deng Xiao-Dong et al., "Isolation and Analysis of Hevein Gene and Its Promoter Sequence," *Acta Botanica Sinica*, 44, 8 (2002): 936-940.
6. A.I. McMullen, "Particulate Ribonucleoprotein Components of Hevea-brasiliensis Latex," *Biochem. J.* 85 (1962):491-495.

7. Jay E. Slater et al., "The Latex Allergen Hev b 5 Transcript Is Widely Distributed after Subcutaneous Injection in BALB/c Mice of Its DNA Vaccine," *J. Allergy Clin. Immunol.* 102 (1998):469-75.

8. H. Breiteneder et al., "Rapid Production of Recombinant Allergens in Nicotiana Benthamiana and Their Impact on Diagnosis and Therapy," *Int. Arch. Allergy Immunol.*, 124, 1-3 (2001):48-50.

9. CDC, "General Recommendations on Immunizations, Recommendations of the Advisory Committee on Immunization Practices (ACIP) and the American Academy of Family Physicians (AAFP)," http://www.cdc.gov/mmwr/preview/mmwrhtml/rr5102a1.htm, accessed 1/11/11.

10. Medline Plus, A service of the U.S. National Library of Medicine - National Institutes of Health, http://www.nlm.nih.gov/medlineplus/latexallergy.html, accessed 1/11/11.

11. AnnArbor.com Staff, March 1, 2010, 1 in 4 parents believes vaccines cause autism, University of Michigan study shows, http://www.cbsnews.com/stories/2010/03/01/health/main6255764.shtml, accessed 1/11/11.

12. Steven Reinberg, "Many American Plan to Skip Flu Shot This Year, HealthDay, http://news.yahoo.com/s/hsn/20101007/hl_hsn/manyamericansplantoskipflushotthisyear, accessed 1/11/11.

13. Vaccine injury table, 42 CFR 100.3, http://cfr.vlex.com/vid/100-3-vaccine-injury-table-19796238, accessed 1/11/11.

─────

Chapter 10

Vaccination
Atopic child so fragile, parents so brave, doctors so giving
Science to study, science to learn
Autism spectrum disorder discern

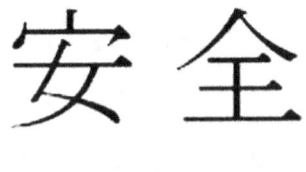

Safety

Safety First

In this Chapter, we'll take a brief look at questions often asked before a child (0-17 years) is immunized and suggest vaccine safety procedure.

It is clear that *Hevea*-allergen contamination in vaccines and subsequent immune sensitivity is unpredictable based on the cleanliness of the natural latex, and the unpredictable characteristics of adaptive immunity. Because the threshold of sensitivity to the *Hevea*-allergens is unknown, it is time for medical science, and government agencies entrusted to assure vaccine safety, to completely abolish the use of *HDNR* in vaccines.

A physician shall, while caring for a patient, regard responsibility to the patient as paramount.[1]

The first question often asked in a vaccination questionnaire is:

Is the child sick today?

The American Heritage® Medical Dictionary defines the term sick as "suffering from or affected with a disease or disorder." It is the authors opinion that medical science needs to use safe and reliable test procedures to answer this question and not rely on a parent's medical expertise. For example, a child does not always show clear signs of being sick and it is understood that a fever may appear several days after being infected.

Another question often asked in immunization screening questionnaires is:

Does the child have allergies to medications, foods, or vaccines?

Again, it is the authors' opinion that it is unreasonable to expect parents to clearly recognize the adverse events associated with allergies in infants. Furthermore, only when *in-vitro* or *in-vivo* allergy tests are run on specific allergens, by medical professionals in certified laboratories, can such a question be answered with confidence. Furthermore, diagnosis of latex allergy is not always straightforward. Several types of tests are currently used. Blood tests for latex allergy have varying levels of reliability. Skin testing for latex allergy is problematic. There is no FDA approved latex-allergen extract available in the U.S. to standardize natural-latex skin testing. Challenge testing may help to clarify latex allergy in ambiguous cases, but both skin and challenge testing run the risk of provoking severe allergic reactions in allergic individuals.[2]

Can vaccines cause acute illness and an adverse event?

According to the CDC and American Academy of Pediatrics (AAP), there is no evidence that acute illness increases vaccine adverse events.[3, 4, 5] In contradiction, the authors suggest that anaphylactic shock associated with atopy falls under the definition of acute illness and can be considered an adverse event.

From a historical perspective, in his presentation speech as winner of the 1913 Nobel Prize in Medicine for his work with anaphylaxis, Charles Robert Richet said, "We are so constituted that we can never receive other proteins into the blood than those that have been modified by digestive juices. Every time alien protein penetrates by effraction, the organism suffers and becomes resistant. This resistance lies in increased sensitivity, a sort of revolt against the second parenteral injection, which would be fatal. At the first injection, the organism was taken by surprise and did not resist. At the second injection, the organism mans its defenses and answers by the anaphylactic shock." In naming "anaphylaxis," Richet described, "Phylaxis, a word seldom used, stands in the Greek for protection. Anaphylaxis will thus stand for the opposite. Anaphylaxis, from its Greek etymological source, therefore, means that state of an organism in which it is rendered hypersensitive, instead of being protected." Richet concluded his lecture by saying, "Seen in these terms, anaphylaxis is a universal defense mechanism against the penetration of heterogeneous substances in the blood, whence they cannot be eliminated."[6]

Where is the wisdom we have lost from knowledge?

The CDC states, "If a person reports a severe (anaphylactic) allergy to latex, vaccines supplied in vials or syringes that contain natural latex should not be administered unless the benefit of vaccination outweighs the risk for a potential allergic reaction. For latex allergies other than anaphylactic allergies (e.g., a history of contact allergy to latex gloves), vaccines supplied in vials or syringes that contain dry natural rubber or rubber latex can be administered."[7, 8]

In 2009, health authorities investigated why a West Australian woman went into anaphylactic shock after receiving the swine flu vaccine. It was suggested that the woman had an allergy to latex, which was present in the bungs of the syringes sent out to doctors with the vaccine.[9]

Thus, it is patently obvious that vaccines that contain HDNR can cause acute illness (i.e., latex allergy) and an adverse event (i.e., anaphylactic shock).

What tests can be run to improve vaccine safety?

In Chapter 11 (Foreseeable Future), specific blood and saliva tests are recommended to help physicians and parents determine if a vaccine should be administered. These tests are intended to measure adaptive-immunity markers (e.g., IgE expression, cytokines, and NGF) to help determine an immunity profile for the child. Children having an 'atypical' adaptive-immunity profile need to be exempt from vaccinations.

Medical science and the general public understand that there is health risks associated with vaccinations. An open and honest discussion about the safety of forced vaccinations must continue. An absolute statement like 'Vaccines do not cause Autism' is intuitively unreasonable based on known adverse-advents associated with vaccinations.

I know that most men—not only those considered clever, but even those who are very clever, and capable of understanding most difficult scientific, mathematical, or philosophic problems—can very seldom discern even the simplest and most obvious truth if it be such as to oblige them to admit the falsity of conclusions they have formed, perhaps with much difficulty—conclusions of which they are proud, which they have taught to others, and on which they have built their lives. – Leo Tolstoy (1828-1910)

_____

Notes

1. AMA Principles of Medical Ethics, "Principle VIII" (Standard of conduct which define the essentials of honorable behavior for a physician), http://www. cirp.org/library/statements/ama/, accessed 1/11/11.
2. Nursing Practice, NYSNA's Education, Latex Allergy, Position Statement, http://www.nysna.org/practice/ positions/position40.htm, accessed 1/11/11.
3. CDC, General recommendations on immunizations, www.cdc.gov/vaccines/pubs/acip-list.htm, accessed 1/11/11.
4. AAP, *2006 Red Book: Report of the Committee on Infectious Diseases, 27th ed.,* (Elk Grove Village, IL: AAP, 2006).
5. Park Nicollet Health Services, Immunization Screening Questionnaire for 0-17 years, 11600 (12/2008).
6. Richet, Charles - Nobel Lecture Dec. 11, 1913, http://www.nobel.se/medicine/laureates/1913/ richet-lecture.html, accessed 1/11/11.
7. CDC, "Latex in Vaccine Packaging," http://www. cdc.gov/vaccines/pubs/pinkbook/downloads/ appendices/B/latex-table.pdf, accessed 1/11/11.
8. Advisory Committee on Immunization Practices (ACIP), General Recommendations on Immunization, http://www.cdc.gov/vaccines/recs/ acip/default.htm, accessed 1/11/11.
9. The Age, "Shock Reaction Sparks Flu Vaccine Inquiry," http://www.theage.com.au/national/ shock-reaction-sparks-flu-vaccine-inquiry-20091007- gn93.html, accessed 1/11/11.

_____

11

Chapter 11

Immunity of life
Pre-vaccination, keeping baby safe from regression
Test before injection
Immunoglobulins in blood, neurotrophin in saliva
Cytokine and androgen expression
Post-vaccination, keeping baby safe from regression
Test after injection
Immunoglobulins in blood, neuron growth factor in saliva
Cytokine expression
Baby Safe from Regression

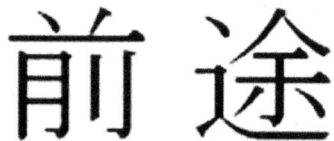

Future

Foreseeable Future

In 1802, Edward Jenner publishes his first results claiming that scratching cowpox pus into the arms of healthy children could protect them against smallpox. Over the years, vaccine safety has improved dramatically but there are still safety questions to be answered.

In *Vaccine Delivery and Autism (The Latex Connection)*, the authors describe how vaccines can cause atopy and allergy-induced regressive autism in immune-sensitive individuals. As a safety measure, a number of vaccine guidelines and procedures are suggested below.

- Eliminate *HDNR* in vaccines.
- Medical research to define an 'atypical' adaptive-immunity profile.
- Require adaptive-immunity test for individuals prior to each vaccination.
- Children having an 'atypical' adaptive-immunity profile (e.g., over-expression of neurotrophin and IgE, skewed cytokine profile) need to be exempt from vaccinations.

Will pre-vaccination testing reduce vaccine injury?

The humoral expression of endogenous proteins including IgE, cytokines, and neurotrophin may affect the safety of forced immunity. Quantifying these proteins in the blood could help determine if a child can be safely vaccinated without inducing an adverse event (e.g., anaphylactic shock, atopy, allergy-induced regressive autism). Described below are scientific studies showing how these proteins affect autism.

Evaluating serum IgE and autism, a study showed that allergy may play a role in the pathogenesis of autism wherein allergic immune responses to some proteins (e.g., dietary proteins and latex) may induce the production of brain autoantibodies, which are found in many autistic children. This study was conducted to investigate the frequency of allergic manifestations in autistic children. The relationship between allergy and disease characteristics in terms of disease severity, clinical findings and electroencephalography (EEG) abnormalities was also studied. Fifty autistic children (30 had mild to moderate autism and 20 had severe autism) were studied in comparison to 50 age- and sex- matched children without neuropsychiatric manifestations serving as controls. Clinical evaluation was done with special emphasis on neuropsychiatric assessment and clinical manifestations of allergy. Serum total IgE was measured in all studied subjects. In addition, EEG and assessment of mental age were done for all autistic children. Allergic manifestations (bronchial asthma, atopic dermatitis and/or allergic rhinitis) were found in 52% of autistic patients. This frequency was significantly higher than that of controls (10%; $P < 0.001$). There was a significant positive association between the frequency of allergic manifestations and disease severity, important clinical findings elicited in some autistic children (gastrointestinal symptoms and neurological manifestations) and EEG abnormalities. The researchers concluded that the frequency of allergic manifestations is increased in autistic children. The significant positive association between these manifestations and important disease characteristics (disease severity, gastrointestinal symptoms, neurological findings and EEG abnormalities) may shed light on the possible causal role of allergy in some autistic children. Indeed, we need to know more about the links between allergy, immune system and brain in autism. This is important to determine whether therapeutic modulation of immune function and allergic diseases are legitimate avenues for novel therapy in selected cases of autism or even for attempted primary prevention in genetically at risk subgroups.[1]

Evaluating cytokines and autism, a study compared production of IL-2, IFN-gamma, IL-4, IL-13, IL-5 and IL-10 in peripheral blood mononuclear cells from 20 children with autism spectrum disorder to those from matched controls. Levels of all T_H2 cytokines were significantly higher in cases after incubation in media alone, but the IFN-gamma/IL-13 ratio was not significantly different between cases and controls. Cases had significantly higher IL-13/IL-10 and IFN-gamma/IL-10 than controls. The researchers concluded that children with ASD had increased activation of both T_H2 and T_H1 arms of the adaptive immune response, with T_H2

predominance, and without the compensatory increase in the regulatory cytokine IL-10.[2]

Could a simple test for NGF be used to determine if a child can be safely vaccinated?

In the future, a simple test may be used to determine if a child can be safely vaccinated.

For example, saliva testing for NGF, before and after vaccinating, could be a useful non-invasive medical procedure to evaluate if a child is experiencing the manifestations of atopy and allergy-induced regressive autism.[3] The expression of NGF could be monitored, especially in the first two years of life, in an effort to reduce neural over-connectivity. If a child has elevated levels of NGF, a vaccine should not be given.

As previously discussed in Chapter 4 (Life Design), the over-expression of NGF during prenatal/neonatal/infant development may affect the neural pruning mechanism, resulting in over-connectivity. As additional evidence, recent studies indicate over-connectivity in ASD. Specifically, a review highlighted neurobiological findings during the first years of life and emphasizes early brain overgrowth as a key factor in the pathobiology of autism. Research showed that excess neuron numbers may be one possible cause of early brain overgrowth and may produce defects in neural patterning and wiring, with exuberant local and short-distance cortical interactions impeding the function of large-scale, long-distance interactions between brain regions. Researchers suggest that because large-scale networks underlie socio-emotional and communication functions, such alterations in brain architecture could relate to the early clinical manifestations of autism.[4]

Why test before we inject?

The Autism Society of America has written, "Despite the lack of prevalence data on autism worldwide, there are emerging trend numbers that suggest that tens of millions of children and adults have ASD. As the numbers increase, the resulting costs of this lifespan condition on national economies rise concurrently; by 2010, estimates of the cost of caring for the estimated 1.75 million Americans with ASD will reach $90 billion per year. In countries such as India, Russia and Nigeria, these costs could cripple a nation's health and education budgets within a few years."[5]

A study estimated the costs of ASD in the UK. Data on prevalence, level of intellectual disability, and place of residence were combined with average annual costs of services and support, together with the opportunity costs of lost productivity. The costs of supporting children with ASDs were estimated to be 2.7 billion each year. For adults, these costs amount to 25 billion each year. The lifetime cost, after discounting, for someone with ASD and intellectual disability is estimated at approximately 1.23 million, and for someone with ASD without intellectual disability is approximately 0.80 million.[6]

The economics of ASD clearly suggests that a change in vaccine safety procedures is imperative. Although the vaccine safety procedures described above will be more expensive, it will protect immune-sensitive individuals and help reduce the incidence of atopy and allergy-induced regressive autism.

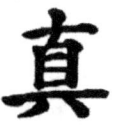

Trust

In the future...

- Medical professionals will do blood tests before and after vaccinations, monitoring adaptive immunity.
- The expression of cytokines, IgE, and NGF will be measured in children to help physicians and parents determine if a vaccine should be administered.

- A child with an "atypical" adaptive immunity profile will be exempt from vaccinations.
- Blood tests will be used to show a biological connection to vaccine injury (i.e., VICP).

Finally, the etiology of vaccine damage is complex. In the spirit of gratitude for the children injured by vaccinations, state-of-the-art allergy intervention and healthcare should be provided for their well-being; let us recognize and honor their sacrifice to defend the health of humanity from infectious disease.

Disabled child, casualty of vaccine
Society indebted
Assimilate
Appreciate
Compensate

The evidence (vaccines cause autism) is now overwhelming, despite the misinformation from the Centers for Disease Control and Prevention, the American Academy of Pediatrics, and the Institute of Medicine. – Bernard Rimland (American Research Psychologist)

Notes

1. Gehan A. Mostafa et al., "Allergic Manifestations in Autistic Children: Relation to Disease Severity, *J. Pediatr. Neurol.* 6, 2 (2008):115-123.
2. CA Molloy et al., "Elevated cytokine levels in children with autism spectrum disorder", *J. Neuroimmunol*, 2006 Mar; 172(1-2):198-205.
3. Eric Courchesne et al., "Mapping Early Brain Development in Autism." *Neuron* 56, 2 (2007): 399-413.

4.   J.K. Nam, J.W. Chung, H.S. Kho, S.C. Chung, et al., "Nerve Growth Factor Concentration in Human Saliva, *Oral Disease* 13, 2 (2007):187-192.

5.   Autism Society of America, Incidence numbers from other countries, http://www.autism-society.org/site/PageServer?pagename=community_world_incidenc, accessed 1/11/11.

6.   Martin Knapp et al., "Economic Cost of Autism in the UK," *Autism* 13, 3 (2009):317-336.

———

12

Chapter 12

High-functioning autism, a gift from Mother Nature
Differences in thought, expression, behavior
Mankind will know
Mankind will savor
Science ~ writing ~ music ~ art
Special honor, attention, and favor
Evolutionary distinction
Do not waiver
~

Low-functioning autism, a mishap of medical science
Regression of thought, expression, behavior
Mankind will inject
Mankind will suspect
Atopy ~neural over-connectivity ~ mental disability
Special care
Forced detention
Reaffirms
Vaccine-safety evolution

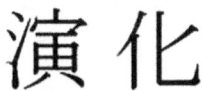

演 化

Evolution

———

Autism Distinction

Allergy-induced autism is part of the evolutionary process for mankind. Within the autism spectrum, some individuals have exceptional cognitive skills in mathematics, music, science, art, and writing. At the same time, these same individual may also have severe and pervasive impairment in thinking, feeling, language, and sociability. This is often referred to as fractured skills.

What is the etiology of fractured skills in autism?

It is speculated that the interaction of environmental insult (allergens) and epigenetics (protein transcription) affects neurological development through atypical adaptive-immunity (atopy). It is further speculated that fractured skills are a result of neural over-connectivity (hard wiring) which facilitates the amplification of certain types of perceptions and focus beyond the level achieved by neuro-typical individuals. The degree of neural over-connectivity, in a region of the brain, can dramatically increase focus in one activity but reduce it in others. As an analogy, a seven lane freeway is created that allows a great number of automobiles to move swiftly and efficiently in and out of a city. The novel freeway is constructed and maintained with such complexity and precision that it is considered state-of-the-art. Maintenance of the freeway consumes an exorbitant amount of resources; secondary roads that lead in and out of the city become neglected and diminish in usefulness. When the secondary roads falter or fail, the over-all flow of traffic will be adversely affected and be considered 'atypical', compared to other cities that have 'typical' roadway infrastructure.

What are some examples of autistic individuals that had unique cognitive skills?

A book written by Michael Fitzgerald, of the Department of Child Psychiatry at Trinity College, Dublin, describes some historical figures with autism. Fitzgerald speculates that the following gifted individuals may have been autistic.

- Writers – Hans Christian Andersen, Lewis Carroll, Bruce Chatwin, Arthur Conan Doyle, Herman Melville, George Orwell, Jonathan Swift, and William Butler Yeats
- Philosophers – A.J. Ayer, Baruch de Spinoza, Immanuel Kant, Simone Weil, and Ludwig Wittgenstein
- Musicians – Bela Bartok, Ludwig van Beethoven, Glenn Gould, Wolfgang Amadeus Mozart, and Erik Satie
- Artists – Vincent van Gogh, L.S. Lowry, Jack B. Yeats, and Andy Warhol[1, 2, 3]
- Scientists – Albert Einstein (1879–1955) and Isaac Newton (1643–1727) may have had Aspergers syndrome[4]

It is evident that high-functioning autism has existed throughout history. At present, there continues to be a long and growing list of exceptionally creative people known or speculated to be diagnosed with autism.[5]

However, many individuals on the autism spectrum have severe and pervasive impairment in thinking, feeling, language, and sociability. It is well documented that there is a disproportionate number of borderline, mild, moderate, severe, and profoundly severe mentally retarded individuals on the autism spectrum. Researchers have proposed that the fraction of autistic individuals who meet criteria for mental retardation has been reported from 25 percent to 70 percent.[6] This large range shows a staggering diversity and uncertainty associated with ASD research.

The CDC states, "CDC estimates that an average of 1 in 110 children in the U.S. has an ASD. The CDC is working to find out how many children have an ASD, discover the risk factors, and raise awareness of the signs."[7]

Elsewhere, it has been proposed that we need to redefine autism as a multi-organ metabolic disease that should be removed from the DSM-IV, placed in the medical textbooks instead, and routinely taught in medical schools and residences.[8]

Has vaccine-insult increased the incidence of mental retardation in allergy-induced regressive autism?

As discussed in previous Chapters, medical research has shown that vaccinations can increase allergy sensitivity. In atopic children, vaccinations could be the tipping point that further induces the prevalence of allergic reactions; adversely affecting cognitive development. It is the opinion of the authors (i.e., Michael J. Dochniak and Denise H. Dunn) that atypical adaptive immunity, and *Hevea*-allergen tainted vaccines, continues to affect the incidence of mental retardation in allergy-induced regressive autism.

The Hevea-allergens *can activate the immune system and adversely change the autistic mind.*
– Michael J. Dochniak

———

Notes

1.   Michael Fitzgerald, *The Genesis of Artistic Creativity: Asperger's Syndrome and the Arts* (London: Jessica Kingsley Publishers, 2005).
2.   Antoinette Walker and Michael Fitzgerald, *Unstoppable Brilliance: Irish Geniuses and Asperger's Syndrome* (Amazon.com: Liberties Press 2006).
3.   Michael Fitzgerald, *Autism and Creativity: Is There a Link between Autism in Men and Exceptional Ability?* (East Sussex: Brunner-Routledge, 2004).

4.   "Historical figures sometimes considered autistic," Wikipedia, The free encyclopedia, http://en.wikipedia.org/wiki/People_speculated_to_have_been_autistic, accessed 1/11/11.

5.   "List of people on the autism spectrum," Wikipedia, The free encyclopedia, http://en.wikipedia.org/wiki/List_of_people_on_the_autism_spectrum, accessed 1/11/11.

6.   M. Dawson et al., "Learning and Memory: A Comprehensive Reference," *Academic Press* (2008):759-72.

7.   Centers for Disease Control and Prevention, "Autism Spectrum Disorders (ASDs)," http://www.cdc.gov/ncbddd/autism/index.html, accessed 1/11/11.

8.   Bryan Jepson and Jane Johnson, *Changing the Course of Autism: A Scientific Approach for Parents and Physicians* (Amazon.com: First Sentient Publications, 2007), 45.

———

13

Chapter 13

Natural latex contaminated vaccine
Complex solution to force immune resolution
Antibody pollution
Memory B cells function, IgE primed mast-cell dysfunction
Multiple allergies within

~

Adaptive immunity, out of control army
Friendly fire begin
Atopy and cross-reactivity
Sensitive to many proteins therein
Autoimmunity and over-connectivity

~

Regressive autism within, if we continue to ignore...
Contaminated- vaccine spin
Failure to adapt
Failure to comprehend
Mankind gets confused, in the mind with time
Earth becomes a prison of tainted vaccines

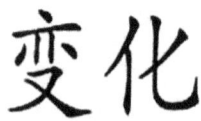

Change

———

The Change

In 2010, the U.S. extended its existing recommendations for routine influenza vaccination to all persons with the exception of infants less than six months of age. Thus, routine influenza vaccination is recommended for all persons six months and older.[1]

Why flu vaccines for Children?

A study showed that the high costs of hospitalizing young children for influenza creates a significant economic burden in the United States, underscoring the importance of preventive flu shots for children and the people with whom they have regular contact. Researchers analyzing data in three U.S. cities over the course of three flu seasons (2003-2006) found that 90 percent of the highest-cost hospitalizations for children were linked to influenza, with a co-infection of the respiratory tract.[2] Influenza is not a major cause of death in children. The majority of deaths from influenza, in the industrialized world, occur in adults at the age of 65 years and older.[3]

In a study published online in *The Journal of the American Medical Association*, researchers reported that the vaccination of school-age children has a strong protective effect on the adults and elderly with whom the children are in contact. Dr. Fauci stated, "Not only was that clearly needed to protect the kids, but they probably wound up protecting the older people, too."[4]

It has been shown that some pharmaceutical companies continue to use *HDNR* in flu vaccines. In 2010, the FDA required label changes for flu vaccines to highlight natural latex concerns. Specifically, the changes reflect concerns that the tip caps of flu vaccine products shipped in prefilled syringes contain natural latex, which can cause allergic reactions in latex-sensitive individuals.[5] In parallel, the authors would suggest the following warning for vaccines that contain *HDNR*. "This vaccine may contain

Hevea-allergens that can cause one or more of the following adverse events: latex allergy; food allergies; atopy; allergy-induced regressive autism; and anaphylactic shock."

Why is HDNR within flu-vaccine packaging and delivery systems?

The pharmaceutical companies that use HDNR need to provide the answer. We know there are synthetic rubber alternatives to HDNR including plastics and silicone rubbers. These alternatives may have diminished price/performance characteristics compared to HDNR.

There is no doubt that vaccinations are an important health and safety initiative, but, it's time to make the change. Based on its poor health and safety characteristics, HDNR should not be a part of vaccines; children continue to get sick from repeated exposure to the *Hevea*-allergens therein. This is supported by the following facts.

- *Hevea*-allergens can never be completely removed from HDNR.
- *Hevea*-allergens from HDNR can leach into vaccines.
- *Hevea*-allergens produce natural-latex allergy.
- Natural-latex allergy causes atopy.
- Atopy induces regressive autism.

Children are not immune to the vaccine learning-curve.

– Michael J. Dochniak

─────

Notes

1. "Prevention and Control of Influenza with Vaccines Recommendations of the Advisory Committee on Immunization Practices (ACIP)," 2010 July 29, 2010 / 59 (Early Release):1-62, http://www.cdc.gov/mmwr/preview/mmwrhtml/rr59e0729a1.htm, accessed 1/11/11.

2. Cincinnati Children's Hospital Medical Center, "Young Children Hospitalized for Flu Associated With Higher Costs and Higher Risk Illness," Study results presented May 4 at the Pediatric Academic Society annual meeting in Honolulu, Hawaii, http://www.prnewswire.com/cgi-bin/ stories.pl?ACCT=109&STORY=/www/story/05-01- 2008/0004804012&EDATE=, accessed 1/11/11.

3. World Health Organization, "Seasonal Influenza," http://www.who.int/mediacentre/factsheets/fs211/ en/index.html, accessed 1/11/11.

4. Donald G. McNeil Jr., "Flu Shots in Children Can Help Community," *The New York Times*, March 9, 2010, http://www.nytimes.com/2010/03/10/ health/10flu.html?_r=1&ref=health, accessed 1/11/11.

5. Malik Wilson, "FDA Warns of Latex Reactions from Flu Vaccines," Vaccine DailyNews.com August 26, 2010, http://vaccinenewsdaily.com/news/214867- fda-warns-of-latex-reactions-from-flu-vaccines, accessed 1/11/11.

———

Resources

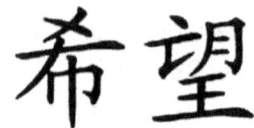

Hope

Every Child by Two, An advocacy organization works to educate parents about vaccines and their safety, http://www.vaccinateyourbaby.org/

Parenting.com: Your Most Common Vaccine Questions, Answered, http://www.parenting.com/article/Child/Health/Your-Most-Common-Vaccine-Questions-Answered

Rubber & Plastics News, organization that describes state of the art rubber news, http://www.rubbernews.com/subscriber/classifieds/rnclass.html

The American Academy of Pediatrics' has a website that provides information on vaccines, up-to-date schedules, safety concerns and the latest vaccine news, http://www.aap.org/immunization/

The Autism Science Foundation provides funding to scientists and organizations conducting, facilitating and promoting autism research, http://www.autismsciencefoundation.org/

The Centers for Disease Control and Prevention's (CDC) comprehensive site, with all the latest news updates, information on each vaccine and recommended schedules, http://www.cdc.gov/

The National Vaccine Injury Compensation Program: 1-800-338-2382, website at http://www.hrsa.gov/vaccinecompensation.

Glossary

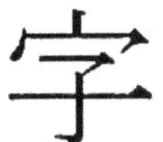

Words

AAFP	American Academy of Family Physicians
AAP	American Academy of Pediatrics
ACIP	Advisory Committee on Immunization Practices
Adaptive immunity	Highly specialized, systemic cells and processes that eliminate or prevent pathogenic challenges
Adjuvant	An immunological agent that modifies the effect of other agents (e.g., vaccines) while having few if any direct effects when given by itself
AIDS	Acquired immune deficiency syndrome; it is the final and most serious stage of HIV disease, which causes severe damage to the immune system.
Allergen	A substance capable of inducing allergy or specific hypersensitivity, such as the natural-latex proteins (Hev-b)
Allergic rhinitis	An allergy affecting the mucus membrane of the nose. Seasonal allergic rhinitis is often called "hay fever."

Allergy	Hypersensitive reaction to a substance harmless to most people
Amino acids	A group of nitrogen-containing chemical compounds that form the basic structural units of proteins
Anaphylaxis	An acute multi-system severe type-I hypersensitivity reaction
Andrew Wakefield	Andrew Wakefield (born 1956) is a British former surgeon and researcher best known for his discredited work regarding the MMR vaccine and its claimed connection with autism and inflammatory bowel disease.
Androgen	Hormones that stimulate male characteristics
Antibody	Proteins manufactured by the body and that bind to an antigen to neutralize, inhibit, or destroy it
Antigen	Any substance that, when introduced into the body, causes the formation of antibodies against it
Arthritis	A group of conditions involving damage to the joints of the body
Asthma	A syndrome caused by chronic inflammation of the airway canal, characterized by increased reactivity of the airways to a variety of stimuli, which results in reversible airway swelling, spasms, and increased mucus production characterized by coughing, wheezing, and shortness of breath.

ASTM	American Society for Testing and Materials
Atopy	A predisposition to various allergic conditions including eczema and asthma
Autoimmune	A process in which antibodies develop against the body's own tissue
Bacteria	A single-celled, microscopic organism existing in many forms, some of which cause disease
Basophile	A type of white blood cell that is involved in allergic reactions
B-cell	The principal functions of B-cells are to make antibodies against antigens
Benign	A medical term used to describe a condition that is harmless
Biochemistry	The chemistry of living organisms
Blood-brain barrier	A special barrier that prevents the passage of materials from the blood to the brain
Brachial neuritis	A sudden onset of shoulder weakness and pain
Chronic	Long-term or frequently recurring
CDC	Centers for Disease Control and Prevention
Cell	The basic subunit of any living organism; the simplest unit that can exist as an independent living system
Class switching	A biological mechanism that changes a B-cell's production of antibody from one class to another
Conjecture	A proposition that is unproven but appears correct and has not been disproven

Comorbidity	The effect of all other diseases or disorders that an individual might have other than the primary disease or disorder of interest
Complex	An aluminum hydroxide-*Hevea*-allergen covalent link or aluminum hydroxide-*Hevea*-allergen hydrogen bonding interaction
Cross-reactivity	The reaction between an antigen and an antibody that was generated against a different but similar antigen
Cytokine	Proteins that are secreted by specific cells of the immune system and glial cells, which carry signals locally between cells, and thus have an effect on other cells
Dementia	Senility; loss of mental function
Dendritic cells (DC)	Immune cells that process antigen material and present it on the surface to other cells of the immune system, thus functioning as antigen-presenting cells; they act as messengers between the innate and adaptive immunity
DNR	Dry natural rubber
Desensitizing	To make (a sensitized or hypersensitive individual) insensitive or nonreactive to a sensitizing agent
EMDT	European Medical Device Technology
Endogenous Protein	A protein coming from inside the body
Encephalopathy	Disorder or disease of the brain

Enzyme	An organic catalyst that speeds chemical reactions
Eosinophil	White blood cells that are one of the immune system components responsible for combating multi-cellular parasites and certain infections in vertebrates
Epigenetics	Changes in phenotype (appearance) or gene expression caused by mechanisms other than changes in the underlying DNA sequence
Estrogens	Hormones that produce female characteristics
Etiology	The study of causation
Exogenous protein	A protein coming from outside the body
FDA	United States Food and Drug Administration
Food allergies	A chronic disease characterized by an overreaction of the immune system to food proteins
Fringe science	Scientific inquiry in an established field of study that departs significantly from mainstream or orthodox theories, and is classified in the "fringes" of a credible mainstream academic discipline
Gene	A sequence of DNA in the nucleus of a cell that codes for the production of a specific protein
HDNR	*Hevea brasiliensis* dry natural latex
Helper T-cell	Lymphocytes that help in the immune response

Herd immunity	A type of immunity that occurs when the vaccination of a portion of the population (or herd) provides protection to unprotected individuals
Hevea brasiliensis	Natural latex from the Para rubber tree
Hev-b	Protein from Para rubber tree
Hevein	An allergenic sugar-binding protein from natural latex
Histamine	A chemical released by basophiles and mast cells that causes nearby tissues to become swollen and inflamed
Hormone	A secretion of an endocrine gland that controls and regulates body function
Hypothesis	A proposed explanation for an observable phenomenon
IgE	Immunoglobulin-E antibody
IgG	Immunoglobulin-G antibody
IgM	Immunoglobulin-M antibody
Immune cells	Cells of the immune system involved in defending the body against both infectious disease and foreign materials
Immunization	A medical treatment that imparts immunity to a specific disease; "vaccinations" and "flu shots" are immunizations
Immunoglobulin-E	A class of antibody (or immunoglobulin "isotype") that has only been found in mammals
Immunoglobulins	Antibodies
Immunomodulation	Changing certain characteristics of the immune system, this may be done as therapy for a disease state

Innate immunity	The cells and mechanisms that defend the host from infection by other organisms
Incidence	The number of new cases of a disease or disorder that occurs during a given period (usually years) in a defined population
Induced	Bring about or give rise to
Inflammation	A fundamental response to injury or abnormal stimulation consisting of complex reactions occurring in the affected blood vessels and adjacent tissues; the inflammatory process includes destruction or removal of the material causing the injury and responses that lead to repair and healing, or responses that lead to a variety of acute and chronic disease states.
Interleukin	Group of cytokines that were first seen to be expressed by white blood cells
In vitro	outside a living body and in an artificial environment
In vivo	in the living body of a person
Latex	An aqueous colloid/emulsion of rubber particles
Latex allergies	A chronic disease characterized by an overreaction of the immune system to latex proteins (Hev-b) found in many natural rubber or latex products; latex allergies may occur due to touching latex or inhaling latex dust.
Leukocyte	White blood cell

Lymphocyte	A type of white blood cell in the vertebrate immune system
Macrophage	Specialized cells that engulf and destroy bacteria and foreign particles in the body
Mast cell	a cell, found in many tissues of the body, that contributes greatly to allergic and inflammatory processes by secreting histamine and other inflammatory particles
Molecule	A specific chemical substance that can exist alone
Natural rubber	The United States Food and Drug Administration terminology for natural rubber latex; rubber obtained from botanical sources
Neurotrophin	A family of proteins that induce the survival, development, and function of neurons
Neutrophil	A white blood cell important in the immune process
Neonate	A human infant less than a month old
Neural pruning	Natural decrease of neural network
Neurotransmitters	Substances that modify or transmit nerve impulses
Neurotrophin	A family of proteins that induce the survival, development, and function of neurons
NGF	Neuron growth factor, a secreted protein that is important for the growth, maintenance, and survival of nerve cells
NINDS	National Institute of Neurological Disorders and Strokes
NIOSH	National Institute of Occupational Safety and Health

NL	Natural latex
NR	Natural rubber
NRL	Natural rubber latex
NVPO	National Vaccine Program Office
OSHA	Occupational Safety and Health Administration, US Department of Labor
Pacifier	A natural-latex nipple given to an infant or other young child to suck on
Para rubber	*Hevea* rubber from uncultivated trees
Pathogen	A biological agent that causes disease to its host
Paul A. Offit	Paul A. Offit, M.D., is an American pediatrician specializing in infectious diseases and an expert on vaccines, immunology, and virology.
Polyisoprene	A polymer component of natural latex
Prenatal	The process in which an embryo or fetus (or *foetus*) gestates during pregnancy, from fertilization until birth.
Preservative	A naturally occurring or synthetic substance that is added to products to prevent decomposition by microbial growth or by undesirable chemical changes
Prevalence	The total number of cases of a disease or disorder in the population at a given time
Prostaglandin	Hormone-like compounds manufactured from essential fatty acids

Proteases Enzymes that degrade other proteins

Proteins Organic compounds made up of amino acids; one of the major constituents of plant and animal cells

Radioallergosorbant A blood test that measures the amount of IgE antibody produced when the sample is mixed with a specific allergen

Receptor In nerves, a specialized nerve ending able to receive and respond to a stimulus in a specific way; used to describe the molecule on a cell surface that interacts with a specific chemical messenger

Regression A characteristic of autism associated with atypical behaviors

Seizure Abnormal excessive or synchronous neuronal activity in the brain

Sepsis The presence of various pus-forming and other pathogenic microorganisms, or their toxins, in the blood

Serum A component of blood

Sequelae A pathological condition resulting from a disease, injury, or other trauma

Skin prick test A test where a needle is used to scratch the skin with a small amount of allergen; a response can usually be seen within 15 to 20 minutes.

Sympathetic-NS One of the three parts of the autonomic nervous system,

	along with the enteric and parasympathetic systems; its general action is to mobilize the body's resources under stress, to induce the fight-or-flight response.
Synaptic pruning	A synonym often used to describe the maturation of behavior and cognitive intelligence in children by "weeding out" the weaker synapses
Sublingual absorption	Under the tongue
Syndrome	A specific set of symptoms and/or medical findings that often occur together but are not distinct enough to be thought of as a single disease entity (e.g., sleep apnea syndrome)
T-cells	Small white blood cells that orchestrate and/or directly participate in the immune defenses; also known as T lymphocytes, they are processed in the thymus and secrete lymphokines.
Testosterone	Hormone that produce male characteristics
The Lancet	*The Lancet* is a weekly peer-reviewed general medical journal
Theory	General principles derived from a body of scientific data to explain a natural occurrence
Thimerosal	An organo-mercury compound established as an antiseptic and antifungal agent
T_H1 and T_H2	A sub-group of lymphocytes that play an important role in

	establishing and maximizing the capabilities of the immune system
Thrombocytopenic	A very low platelet count that can lead to bruises, or more
purpura	seriously, bleeding diathesis
Toxicity	Ability to cause harm
Vaccine	A biological preparation that improves immunity to a particular disease
Virus	A tiny infectious agent that requires a host cell in order to replicate; it is composed of either RNA or DNA wrapped in a protein coat; viruses cause a wide variety of diseases.
WHO	World Health Organization

———

Bibliography

Michael J. Dochniak is a noted writer, speaker, inventor, and author.

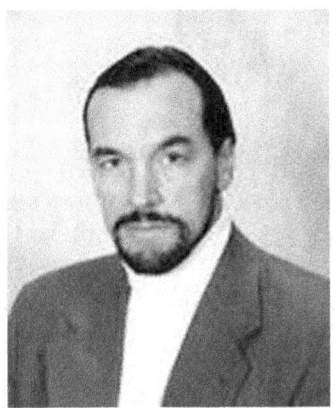

Michael J. Dochniak

Denise Harmony Dunn is an early childhood educator and autism researcher.

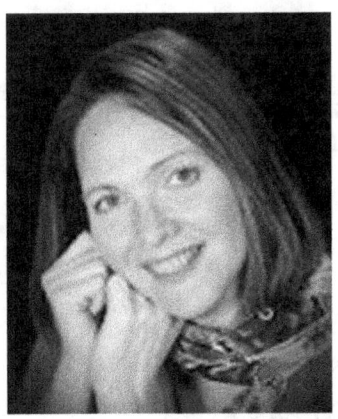

Denise Harmony Dunn

Index

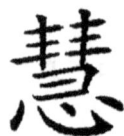

Wisdom